The Complete Acid Reflux Diet Cookbook

Manage GERD & LPR Naturally with Over 110 Healthy, Delicious & Easy Recipes for Better Digestion & Comfort | Includes a Heartburn-Free 30-Day Meal Plan for Lasting Relief

Indulge in Wellness: Where Flavor Meets Healthful Living

Andrew Moore

Legal & Disclaimer

The content and information contained in this book has been compiled from reliable sources, which are accurate based on the knowledge, belief, expertise and information of the Author. The author cannot be held liable for any omissions and/or errors.

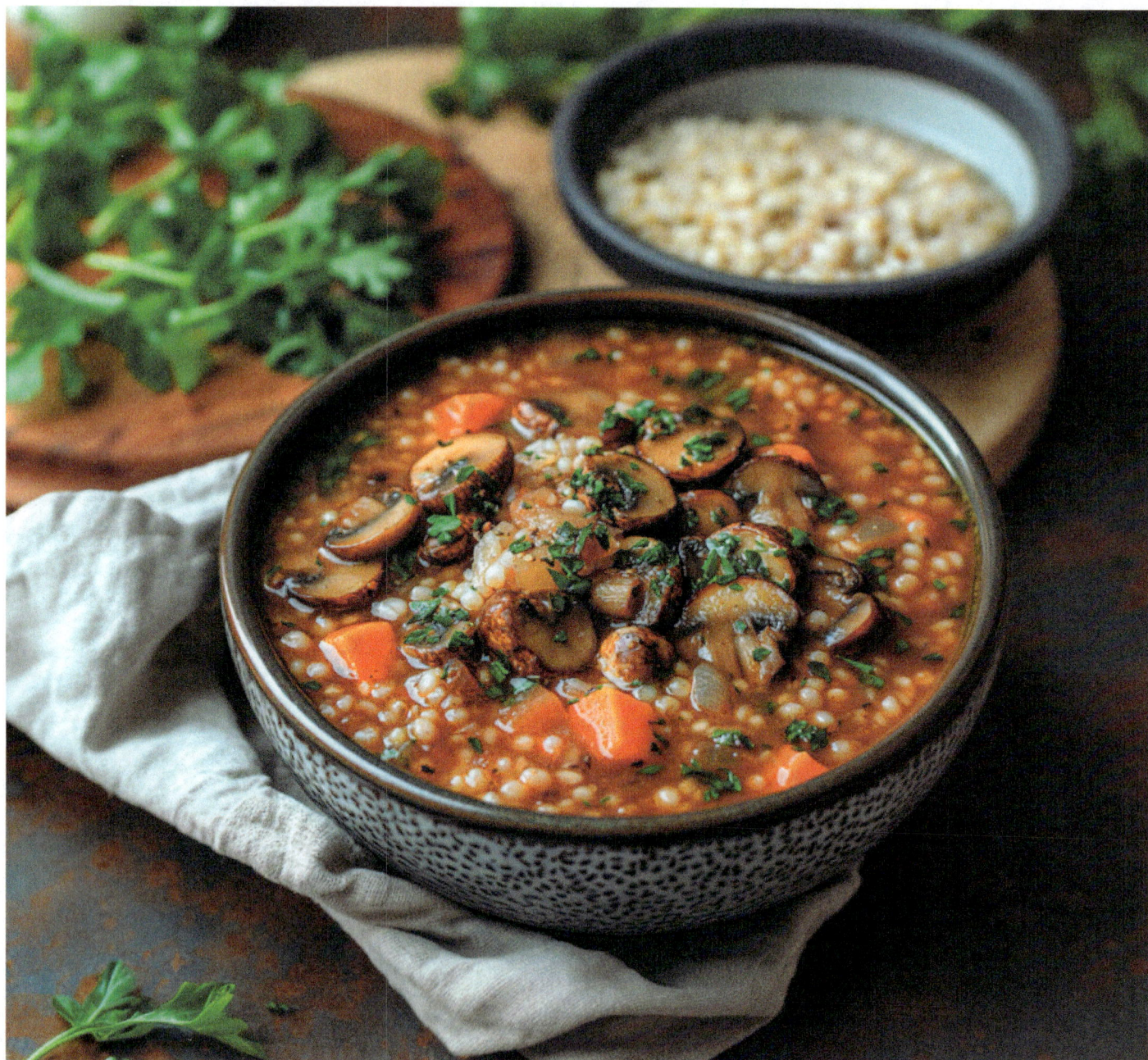

TABLE OF CONTENTS

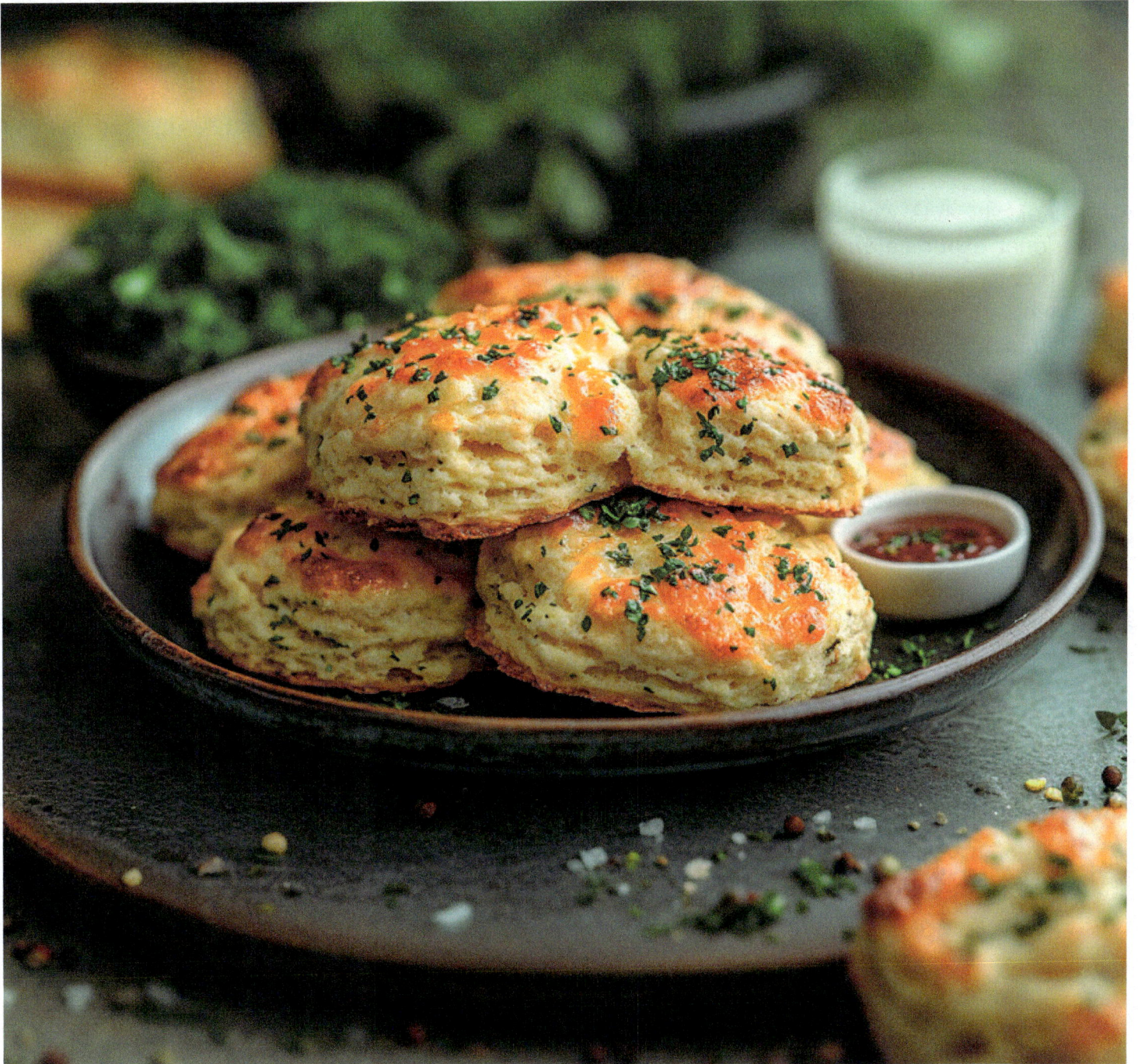

INTRODUCTION

Dear readers,

Andrew Moore, a professional chef renowned for his expertise in creating digestion-friendly cuisine, invites you to explore the world of flavorful, health-conscious cooking with his latest book, *The Complete Acid Reflux Diet Cookbook*. With years of experience in the culinary arts and a deep understanding of GERD, LPR, and acid reflux management, Andrew is a trusted authority in the field of therapeutic cooking.

Andrew's recipes are thoughtfully designed to balance flavor, nutrition, and relief, ensuring that each dish not only soothes symptoms of acid reflux but also delights the palate. His innovative approach focuses on low-acid, easy-to-digest meals that fit seamlessly into a busy lifestyle, making healthy eating simple and accessible.

As a chef who has worked closely with clients managing digestive issues, Andrew combines his professional expertise with practical insights. He understands the challenges of maintaining a diet that supports digestive health while still enjoying food, and his recipes reflect a perfect harmony of these needs. Each dish is crafted to minimize common triggers and promote comfort, helping readers reclaim their joy in eating.

The Complete Acid Reflux Diet Cookbook is more than just a collection of recipes; it's a comprehensive guide to improving digestive health naturally. With over 110 recipes and a 30-day meal plan, Andrew provides readers with the tools and confidence to transition to a heartburn-free lifestyle. From breakfast to dinner, every meal is tailored to soothe and nourish, making the journey to better digestion both delicious and sustainable.

Andrew's passion for helping others shines through every page of this book. His mission is to empower readers to take control of their health through mindful eating and practical cooking strategies. With his guidance, *The Complete Acid Reflux Diet Cookbook* becomes an invaluable resource for anyone seeking relief, balance, and enjoyment at the table.

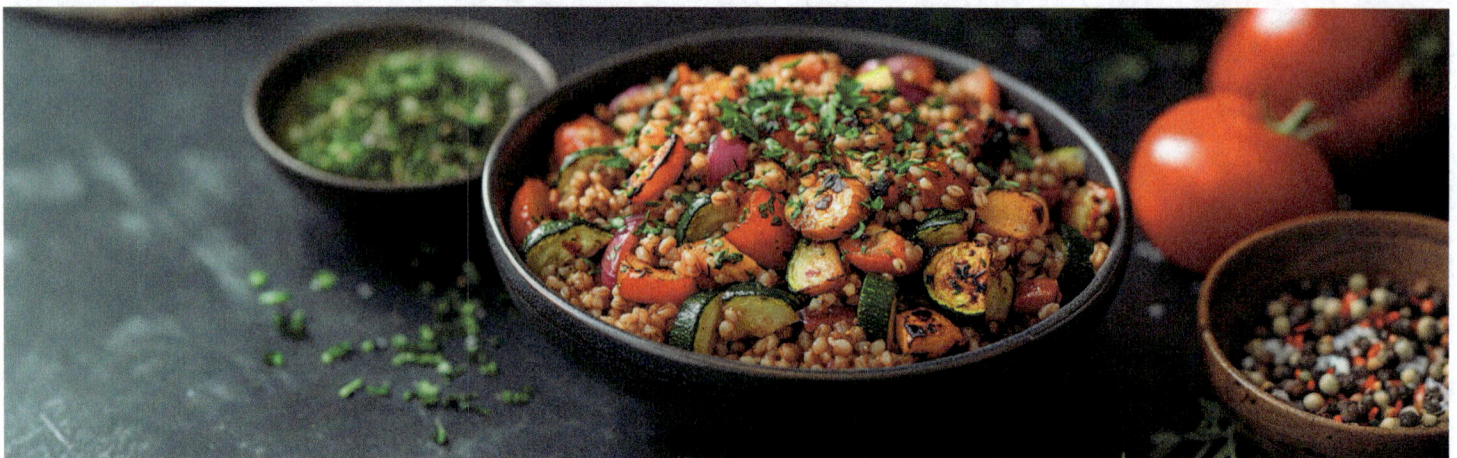

CHAPTER 1: MASTERING THE ACID REFLUX DIET

Understanding the Science Behind Acid Reflux

Acid reflux occurs when stomach acid flows back into the esophagus, causing symptoms like heartburn, a sour taste in the mouth, and discomfort in the chest or throat. GERD is a chronic form of acid reflux, while LPR often affects the throat and voice box. While these conditions can disrupt daily life, they are often influenced by dietary choices and habits.

Key triggers of acid reflux include:

- **Highly acidic foods:** Tomatoes, citrus fruits, and vinegar-based products.
- **Fatty or fried foods:** They relax the lower esophageal sphincter (LES), allowing acid to escape.
- **Spicy ingredients:** Chili, hot sauce, and similar items can irritate the esophagus.
- **Caffeine and carbonated beverages:** These can increase acidity and pressure in the stomach.

By understanding how certain foods and behaviors impact your digestive system, you can take actionable steps toward relief. This isn't about deprivation—it's about choosing foods that work with your body, not against it.

Benefits of an Acid Reflux-Friendly Diet

Switching to an acid reflux-friendly diet has transformative potential for your health and quality of life. Here's what you can expect:

1. Reduced Symptoms and Improved Comfort

By avoiding trigger foods and incorporating low-acid, easy-to-digest ingredients, you can significantly minimize the burning sensation and discomfort of acid reflux.

2. Better Digestive Health

Foods rich in fiber and low in fat, like whole grains, lean proteins, and non-acidic vegetables, promote smoother digestion and reduce the likelihood of reflux.

3. Sustainable Weight Management

Excess weight can contribute to acid reflux by increasing pressure on the stomach. Following this diet can naturally support a healthy weight, further alleviating symptoms.

4. Delicious, Satisfying Meals

An acid reflux diet isn't about bland or boring food. It's about discovering creative ways to enjoy meals that nourish your body while avoiding discomfort. You'll find that flavorful combinations, fresh ingredients, and smart substitutions can make every bite a delight.

What's Ahead

In the chapters to come, we'll dive into a variety of recipes crafted specifically for those managing acid reflux. From soothing breakfasts to hearty dinners and even indulgent desserts, this cookbook offers something for every meal of the day. You'll also find a 30-day meal plan to make your transition seamless and stress-free, along with practical shopping guides to simplify your journey.

You're about to embark on a path to better digestion, improved health, and rediscovered enjoyment of food.

What Is Acid Reflux? Symptoms and Causes

Acid reflux, commonly referred to as heartburn, is more than just a minor inconvenience after a meal. It's a condition that arises when stomach acid flows backward into the esophagus, leading to symptoms that range from mildly uncomfortable to disruptive. Understanding what's happening in your body is the first step to managing acid reflux effectively.

Symptoms of Acid Reflux

The most common symptoms include:

- **Heartburn:** A burning sensation in the chest, often after eating or lying down.
- **Regurgitation:** A sour or bitter taste from stomach acid reaching the throat or mouth.
- **Burping or bloating:** Accompanied by a feeling of fullness.
- **Sore throat or hoarseness:** Often related to LPR (silent reflux).

If acid reflux becomes chronic, it can develop into GERD (Gastroesophageal Reflux Disease), which may cause long-term damage to the esophagus if left untreated.

Causes of Acid Reflux

While triggers vary from person to person, the most common causes include:

1. **Relaxed Lower Esophageal Sphincter (LES):** The LES is a muscle that acts as a barrier between the stomach and esophagus. When it weakens, stomach acid can escape upward.
2. **Certain Foods and Drinks:** Spicy, fatty, and acidic foods, as well as caffeine and alcohol, are known culprits.
3. **Lifestyle Factors:** Overeating, eating close to bedtime, smoking, and stress can all exacerbate reflux.
4. **Excess Weight:** Pressure on the stomach from abdominal fat can push acid upward.
5. **Medical Conditions:** Pregnancy, hiatal hernias, and certain medications can also increase the risk of reflux.

Recognizing the underlying causes and triggers is essential for crafting a diet and lifestyle plan that brings relief.

How Diet Influences Acid Reflux: Myths and Facts

It's no secret that what you eat has a direct impact on acid reflux. But with so much conflicting advice available, it can be challenging to separate fact from fiction. Let's dispel some common myths and focus on the facts about diet and acid reflux.

Myth 1: All Fat Is Bad for Acid Reflux

Fact: While high-fat meals can relax the LES and slow digestion, not all fats are harmful. Healthy fats from sources like avocados (in moderation), olive oil, and nuts can be part of a reflux-friendly diet when consumed in small portions.

Myth 2: Spices Always Trigger Acid Reflux

Fact: Not all spices are created equal. While hot spices like chili and cayenne can irritate the esophagus, milder herbs like basil, parsley, and ginger can be soothing and add flavor to your meals.

Myth 3: All Acidic Foods Are Off-Limits

Fact: Foods with a high acid content, such as tomatoes and citrus fruits, can trigger reflux for some people. However, not everyone reacts the same way. It's about identifying your personal triggers and adjusting accordingly.

Myth 4: Skipping Meals Can Prevent Reflux

Fact: Going long periods without eating can lead to overeating later, which increases the risk of reflux. Instead, focus on smaller, frequent meals to maintain steady digestion and reduce the chance of acid buildup.

The Role of an Acid Reflux-Friendly Diet

A diet tailored to managing acid reflux works by:

1. **Minimizing Triggers:** Avoiding foods that relax the LES or irritate the esophagus.
2. **Promoting Digestion:** Including foods that are easy to digest and help the stomach empty efficiently.
3. **Balancing Acidity:** Focusing on low-acid ingredients that won't exacerbate symptoms.

By understanding how diet impacts your symptoms, you can make informed choices that not only alleviate discomfort but also support your overall health.

Essential Foods for Managing Acid Reflux

When managing acid reflux, the key to success is choosing foods that soothe rather than irritate the digestive system. These foods not only help prevent flare-ups but also provide the nutrition your body needs to thrive. Here's a breakdown of essential foods that should become staples in your kitchen:

Low-Acid Fruits and Vegetables

- **Fruits:** Bananas, melons (honeydew, cantaloupe), apples (sweet varieties, peeled), and pears.
- **Vegetables:** Broccoli, zucchini, spinach, green beans, carrots, and asparagus.

Lean Proteins

- Skinless chicken and turkey.
- Fish such as cod, haddock, and tilapia.
- Egg whites and plant-based proteins like tofu.

Whole Grains

- Oatmeal, quinoa, brown rice, and whole-grain bread (without acidic additives).
- These grains absorb stomach acid and promote digestive health.

Healthy Fats (in moderation)

- Avocado (small portions), olive oil, and flaxseed oil.

- Nuts like almonds and walnuts (handful-sized portions).

Soothing Additions

- **Ginger:** A natural anti-inflammatory that aids digestion.
- **Chamomile tea:** Calms the stomach.

Ingredient Substitution Guide

Cooking for acid reflux doesn't mean giving up flavor. By using smart ingredient substitutions, you can still enjoy a variety of dishes while avoiding triggers.

Trigger Ingredient	Reflux-Friendly Substitute
Tomato sauce	Blended roasted red peppers or carrot-based sauce.
Citrus juice	Cucumber or melon-infused water for acidity-free flavor.
Full-fat dairy	Low-fat milk, almond milk, or oat milk.
Spicy seasonings	Fresh herbs like basil, dill, or parsley.
Fried foods	Baked, grilled, or air-fried alternatives.

These substitutions allow you to create meals that are both safe and satisfying, ensuring you never feel deprived.

Meal Frequency and Portion Control

Eating habits play a significant role in managing acid reflux. Even the healthiest foods can cause discomfort if consumed inappropriately.

Best Practices for Meal Frequency and Portions:

1. **Small, Frequent Meals:** Aim for 4–6 smaller meals or snacks throughout the day rather than three large meals.
2. **Avoid Overeating:** Overfilling your stomach increases pressure on the LES (lower esophageal sphincter), leading to reflux.
3. **Slow Down:** Eat mindfully and chew thoroughly to give your stomach time to process food.
4. **Timing Matters:** Avoid eating within 2–3 hours of bedtime to prevent nighttime reflux.

Acid and Alkaline Food Chart

Balancing acid and alkaline foods can help reduce symptoms. While not all acidic foods cause reflux, prioritizing low-acid, alkaline options is a safe approach.

Food Group	Low-Acid/Alkaline Options	High-Acid Foods to Limit
Fruits	Melons, bananas, pears	Citrus fruits, pineapples
Vegetables	Broccoli, zucchini, spinach	Tomatoes, onions
Proteins	Chicken, turkey, tofu	Fatty cuts of beef, processed meats
Grains	Oatmeal, quinoa, whole-grain bread	Refined white bread, pasta

This chart is a handy reference for planning meals that are aligned with your dietary goals.

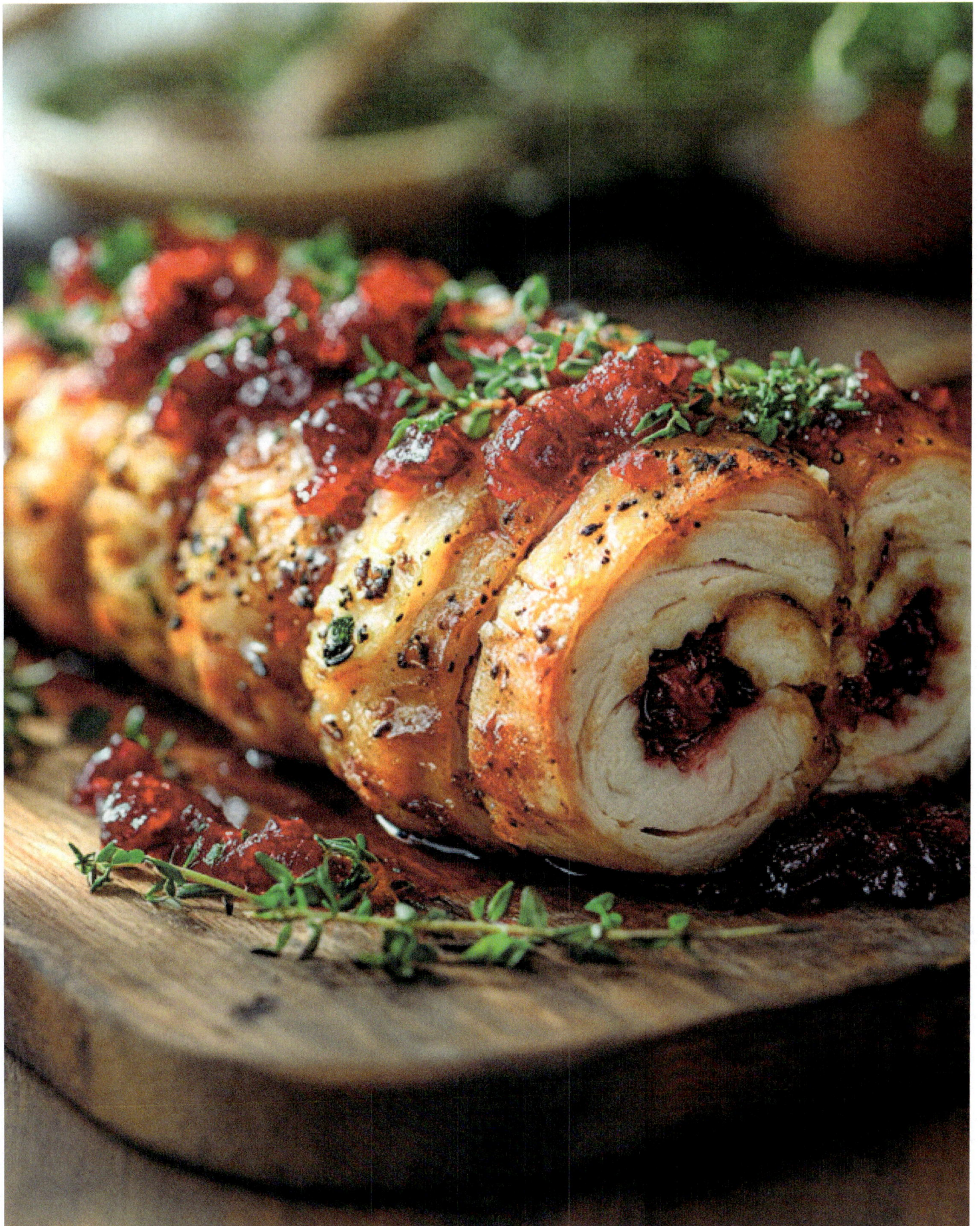

CHAPTER 2: 30-DAY MEAL PLAN

Day	Breakfast	Lunch	Snack	Dinner
Day 1	Oatmeal Honey Muffins - p.15	Creamy Cauliflower Soup - p.29	Ricotta and Herb-Stuffed Eggs - p.45	Stuffed Eggplants Baked with Cheese Crust - p.59
Day 2	Spinach and Ricotta Pancakes - p.17	Pumpkin Sage Pasta - p.33	Apple and Cinnamon Yogurt Dip - p.47	Poached Salmon with Dill Sauce - p.64
Day 3	Pear Ginger Oatmeal - p.18	Chickpea and Quinoa Pilaf - p.36	Mini Chicken Meatballs - p.44	Chicken and Spinach Zucchini Noodle Bake - p.67
Day 4	Egg Casserole with Chicken and Broccoli - p.23	Minestrone Soup - p.32	Herb Cream Cheese - p.48	Vegetable Lasagna with Zucchini Noodles - p.69
Day 5	Pancakes with Cottage Cheese, Vanilla, and Raisins with Yogurt Sauce - p.17	Herb Chicken Pasta Primavera - p.34	Kiwi and Chia Seed Parfait - p.50	Braised Lamb with Rosemary and Vegetables - p.42
Day 6	Kiwi and Spinach Smoothie - p.27	Turkey Meatballs with Spaghetti Squash - p.38	Pumpkin and Sage Spread - p.48	Warm Brussels Sprouts and Bacon Salad - p.58
Day 7	Cabbage Strudel - p.24	Quinoa and Vegetable Stew - p.32	Blueberry and Almond Energy Bites - p.49	Baked Trout with Almonds - p.66
Day 8	Vanilla Chia and Flax Porridge - p.20	Pea and Parmesan Risotto - p.34	Turkey and Cranberry Pinwheels - p.44	Grilled Vegetable Fajitas with Cashew Cheese Sauce - p.62
Day 9	Scrambled Eggs with Zucchini - p.22	Lamb Chops with Sweet Potato Mash - p.39	Spinach and Artichoke Dip - p.46	Haddock Cutlets with Cabbage Salad and Cheese Sauce - p.65
Day 10	Pumpkin Spice Waffles - p.15	Farro and Roasted Vegetable Bowl - p.36	Cakes with Whipped Cottage Cheese Mousse and Seasonal Berries - p.49	Stuffed Pork Tenderloin - p.68
Day 11	Cottage Cheese with Seasonal Berries and Sour Cream Sauce - p.22	Green Pea and Basil Soup - p.30	Basil and Ricotta Spread - p.47	Cauliflower and Lentil Shepherd's Pie - p.61
Day 12	Thin Egg Pancakes with Vegetable Filling - p.23	Spinach and Artichoke Risotto - p.35	Eggs Baked in Small Buns with Bell Peppers - p.43	Grilled Mackerel with Cucumber Salad - p.65
Day 13	Maple Pecan Quinoa Porridge - p.19	Turkey and Wild Rice Soup - p.29	Low-Acid American Popovers - p.55	Roasted Brussels Sprouts with Balsamic Glaze - p.61
Day 14	Spinach and Mushroom Stuffed Chicken Breast - p.25	Mushroom Barley Stew - p.31	Mini Chicken Meatballs - p.44	Mediterranean Chicken Wrap - p.25
Day 15	Kiwi Poppy Seed Waffles - p.16	Amaranth Veggie Patties - p.37	Pumpkin and Coconut Pudding - p.51	Herb-Roasted Turkey with Vegetables - p.42
Day 16	Egg White and Vegetable Wrap - p.21	Pumpkin and Sage Mashed Soup - p.30	Low-Acid Banana Cake - p.54	Fish Lettuce Wraps with Cabbage Slaw - p.64
Day 17	Bruschetta with Boiled Eggs, Soft Cheese, and Asparagus - p.26	Honey Mustard Chicken with Roasted Brussels Sprouts - p.40	Low-Acid Twinkies - p.53	Grilled Vegetable Fajitas with Cashew Cheese Sauce - p.62

Day	Breakfast	Lunch	Snack	Dinner
Day 18	Turkey Sausage and Egg Muffins - p.16	Herb Chicken Pasta Primavera - p.34	Spinach and Feta Stuffed Mushrooms - p.45	Shrimp and Avocado Salad - p.57
Day 19	Blueberries Vanilla Millet Porridge - p.20	Mushroom and Asparagus Risotto - p.35	Turkey and Cranberry Pinwheels - p.44	Chicken and Grape Salad - p.58
Day 20	Cucumber and Apple Smoothie - p.28	Chickpea and Quinoa Pilaf - p.36	Ricotta and Herb-Stuffed Eggs - p.45	Zucchini Noodles with Pesto - p.59
Day 21	Spinach and Ricotta Pancakes - p.17	Minestrone Soup - p.32	Herb Cream Cheese - p.48	Poached Salmon with Dill Sauce - p.64
Day 22	Banana Almond Buckwheat Porridge - p.18	Lean Beef and Lamb Meatloaf with Herbs and Vegetables - p.39	Low-Acid Chelsea Buns - p.53	Grilled Vegetable Fajitas with Cashew Cheese Sauce - p.62
Day 23	Baked Mushroom Fritters with Sour Cream Sauce - p.26	Quinoa and Vegetable Stew - p.32	Kiwi and Chia Seed Parfait - p.50	Warm Brussels Sprouts and Bacon Salad - p.58
Day 24	Pumpkin Spice Waffles - p.15	Asian-Style Boiled Lenten Beef and Broccoli with Wild Rice - p.40	Mini Chicken Meatballs - p.44	Stuffed Calamari with Spinach-Lemon Dressing - p.66
Day 25	Egg White and Vegetable Wrap - p.21	Green Pea and Basil Soup - p.30	Spinach and Artichoke Dip - p.46	Turkey and Spinach Mini Rolls - p.41
Day 26	Vanilla Chia and Flax Porridge - p.20	Farro and Roasted Vegetable Bowl - p.36	Cakes with Whipped Cottage Cheese Mousse and Seasonal Berries - p.49	Cauliflower Rice Bake - p.60
Day 27	Kiwi and Spinach Smoothie - p.27	Herb Chicken Pasta Primavera - p.34	Low-Acid American Popovers - p.55	Stuffed Eggplants Baked with Cheese Crust - p.59
Day 28	Egg Casserole with Chicken and Broccoli - p.23	Pumpkin and Sage Mashed Soup - p.30	Apple and Cinnamon Yogurt Dip - p.47	Chicken and Mushroom Casserole - p.68
Day 29	Maple Pecan Quinoa Porridge - p.19	Turkey Meatballs with Spaghetti Squash - p.38	Mini Chicken Meatballs - p.44	Vegetable Paella - p.62
Day 30	Cottage Cheese with Seasonal Berries and Sour Cream Sauce - p.22	Spinach and Artichoke Risotto - p.35	Blueberry and Almond Energy Bites - p.49	Fish Lettuce Wraps with Cabbage Slaw - p.64

Note: The 30-day meal plan provided in this book is intended as a starting point and a source of inspiration for creating delicious and satisfying meals. Please keep in mind that the caloric and macronutrient values listed for each recipe are approximate and may vary depending on the specific ingredients and portion sizes you use. This plan has been carefully designed to offer a diverse selection of meals that emphasize high-quality proteins and healthy fats while reducing carbohydrates to align with the principles of a ketogenic diet. The goal is to provide a nourishing and flavorful approach to eating every day.

If the portion sizes or calorie estimates don't align perfectly with your unique dietary requirements, feel free to make adjustments. You can easily scale the recipes up or down to better suit your health objectives and personal preferences. This cookbook is crafted to inspire flexibility and creativity in the kitchen, empowering you to enjoy meals that fit your lifestyle while supporting your goals.

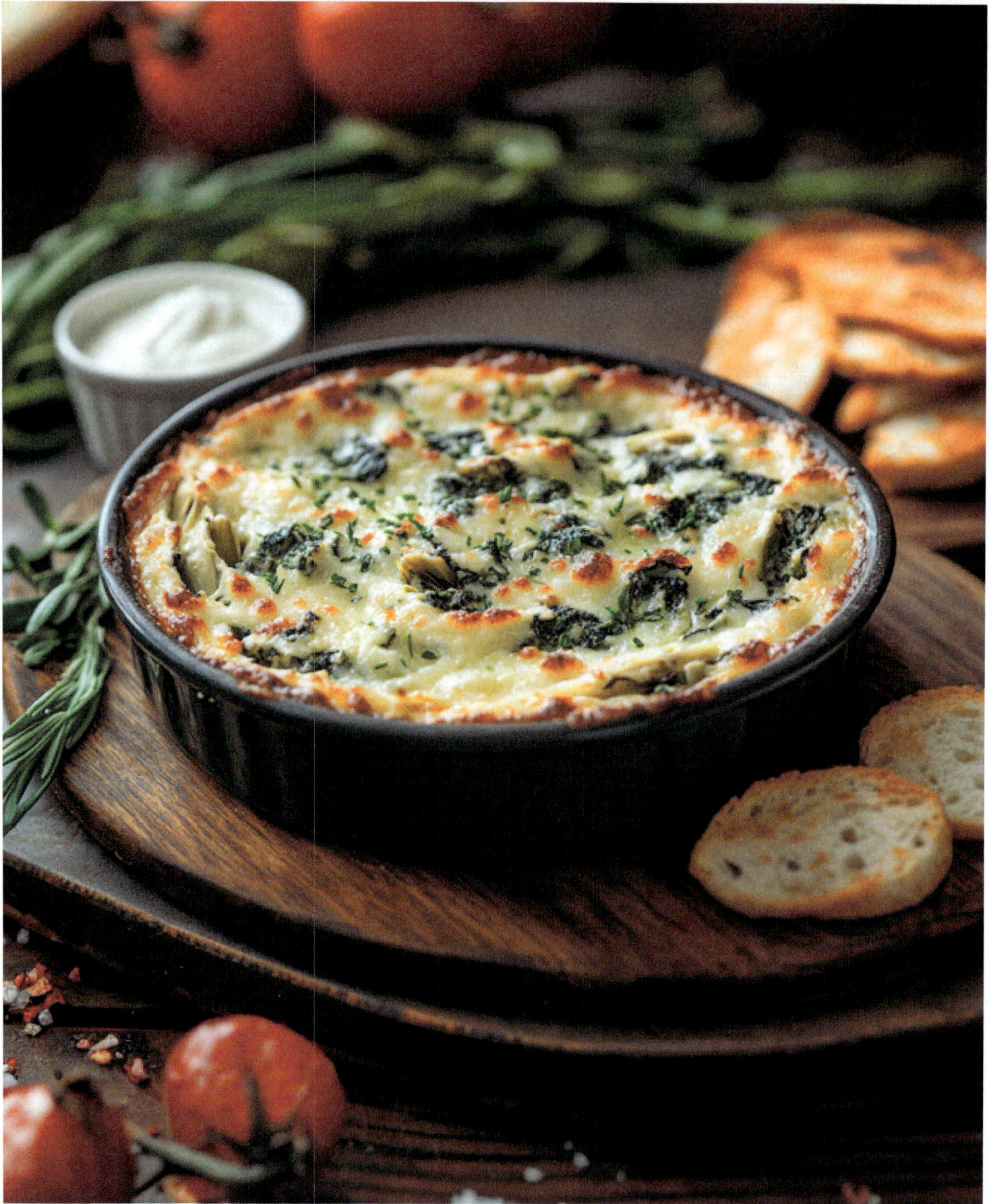

CHAPTER 3: BREAKFASTS:
Low-Acid pancakes, waffles and muffins

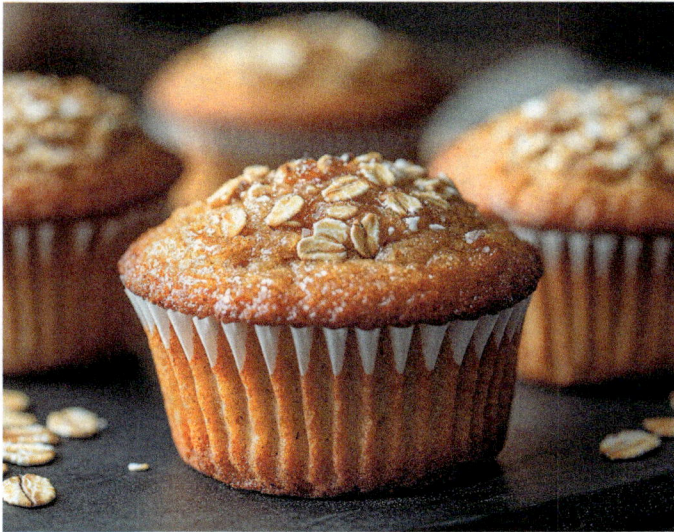

Oatmeal honey muffins

Prep: 10 minutes | Cook: 20 minutes | Serves:4

Ingredients:

- 1 cup rolled oats (90g)
1/2 cup whole wheat flour (60g)
- 1/2 cup almond flour (60g)
- 1 tsp baking powder
- 1/2 tsp baking soda
- 1/4 tsp cinnamon
- 1/4 cup honey (85g)
- 1/2 cup low-fat yogurt (120g)
- 1/4 cup unsweetened applesauce (60g)
- 1 large egg
- 1/2 tsp vanilla extract
- 1/4 tsp salt

Instructions:

1. Preheat the oven to 350°F (175°C) and line a muffin tin with paper liners.
2. In a bowl, combine oats, whole wheat flour, almond flour, baking powder, baking soda, cinnamon, and salt.
3. In another bowl, whisk honey, yogurt, applesauce, egg, and vanilla extract.
4. Mix wet ingredients into the dry mixture until combined.
5. Spoon the batter into muffin liners and bake for 20 minutes or until golden and a toothpick comes out clean.
6. Cool slightly before serving.

Nutritional Facts (Per Serving): Calories: 402 | Protein: 16g | Fat: 14g | Carbs:52 g | Fiber: 7g | Sodium: 760mg | Sugars: 12g

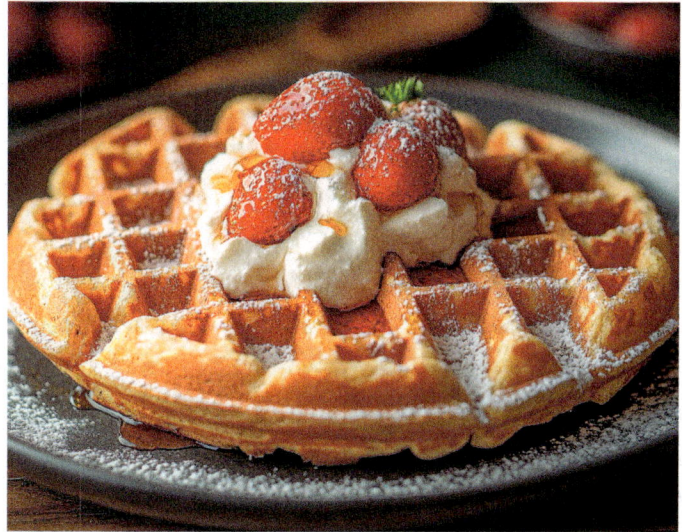

Pumpkin spice waffles

Prep: 10 minutes | Cook: 15 minutes | Serves:4

Ingredients:

- 1 cup whole wheat flour (120g)
- 1/2 cup oat flour (60g)
- 1 tsp baking powder
- 1/2 tsp baking soda
- 1 tsp pumpkin spice
- 1/4 tsp salt
- 1/2 cup pumpkin puree (120g)
- 1/4 cup honey (85g)
- 1/2 cup almond milk (120ml)
- 2 large eggs
- 1 tbsp coconut oil, melted (15g)
- 1 tsp vanilla extract

Instructions:

1. Preheat your waffle iron and lightly grease it with coconut oil.
2. In a large bowl, mix whole wheat flour, oat flour, baking powder, baking soda, pumpkin spice, and salt.
3. In another bowl, whisk pumpkin puree, honey, almond milk, eggs, coconut oil, and vanilla extract.
4. Add wet ingredients to dry ingredients and mix until combined.
5. Pour the batter into the waffle iron and cook for about 5 minutes until golden and crisp.
6. Serve with fresh fruit or a light drizzle of honey.

Nutritional Facts (Per Serving): Calories: 378 | Protein: 18g | Fat: 13g | Carbs: 55g | Fiber: 6g | Sodium: 780mg | Sugars: 10g

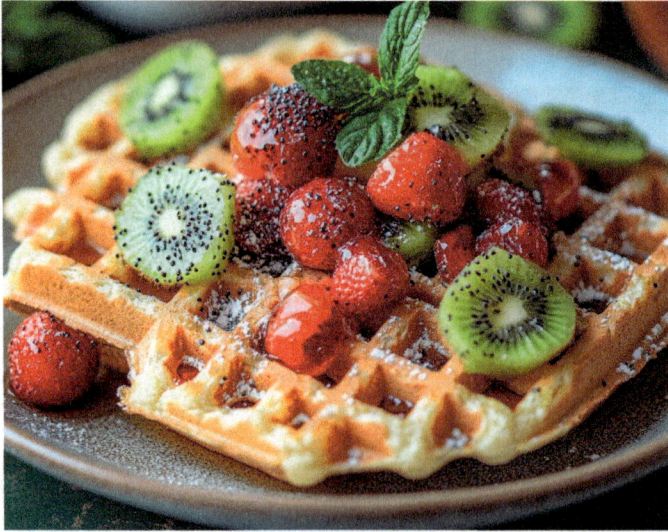

Kiwi poppy seed waffles

Prep: 10 minutes | Cook: 15 minutes | Serves: 4

Ingredients:

- 1 cup oat flour (120g)
- 1/2 cup almond flour (60g)
- 1 tsp baking powder
- 1/4 tsp baking soda
- 1 tbsp poppy seeds (9g)
- 1/4 tsp salt
- 1/4 cup honey (85g)
- 1/2 cup low-fat yogurt (120g)
- 2 large eggs
- 1/2 cup mashed kiwi (120g)
- 1 tbsp coconut oil, melted (15g)
- 1 tsp vanilla extract

Instructions:

1. Preheat the waffle iron and grease it lightly with coconut oil.
2. In a bowl, combine oat flour, almond flour, baking powder, baking soda, poppy seeds, and salt.
3. In another bowl, whisk honey, yogurt, eggs, mashed kiwi, coconut oil, and vanilla extract.
4. Mix wet ingredients into the dry ingredients until smooth.
5. Pour the batter into the waffle iron and cook for 5 minutes or until golden brown.
6. Serve with sliced kiwi or a light drizzle of honey.

Nutritional Facts (Per Serving): Calories: 397 | Protein: 17g | Fat: 14g | Carbs: 57g | Fiber: g | Sodium: 750mg | Sugars: 10g

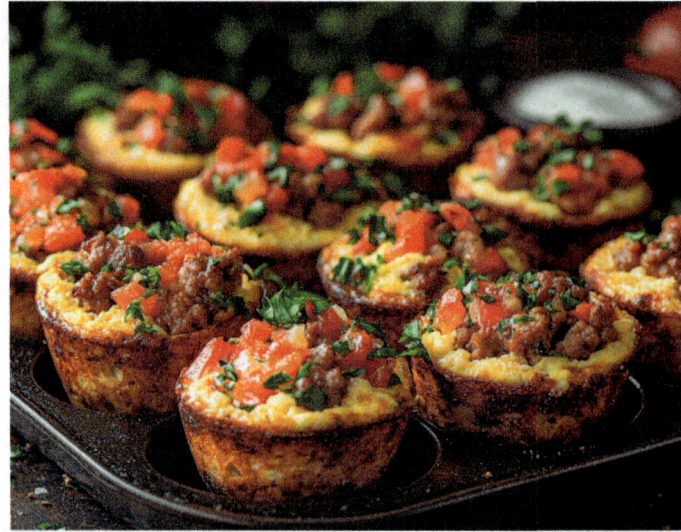

Turkey sausage and egg muffins

Prep: 10 minutes | Cook: 20 minutes | Serves: 4

Ingredients:

- 8 oz ground turkey sausage (225g)
- 6 large eggs
- 1/4 cup almond milk (60ml)
- 1/2 cup bell peppers, diced (75g)
- 1/4 cup onion, diced (30g)
- 1/4 tsp black pepper
- 1/4 tsp salt
- 1/4 tsp garlic powder

Instructions:

1. Preheat oven to 350°F (175°C) and grease a muffin tin.
2. Cook turkey sausage in a pan until browned, then set aside.
3. In a bowl, whisk eggs, almond milk, bell peppers, onion, black pepper, salt, and garlic powder.
4. Stir in the cooked turkey sausage.
5. Pour the mixture evenly into the muffin tin and bake for 20 minutes or until set.
6. Let cool slightly before serving.

Nutritional Facts (Per Serving): Calories: 387 | Protein: 22g | Fat: 15g | Carbs: 56g | Fiber: 5g | Sodium: 780mg | Sugars: 8g

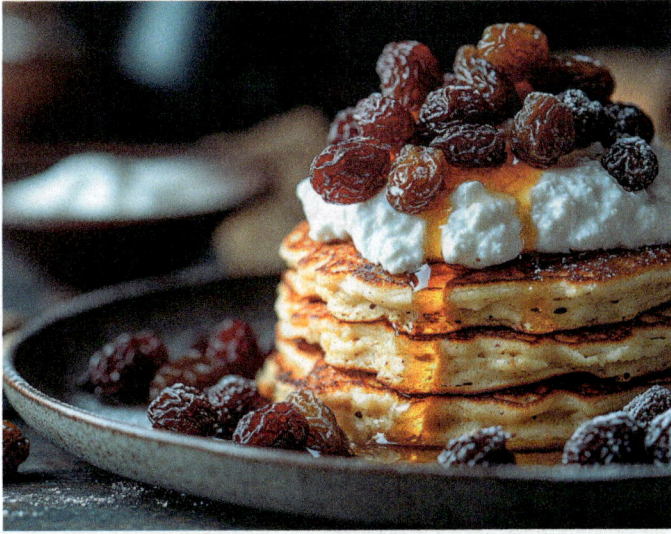

Pancakes with cottage cheese, vanilla, and raisins with yogurt sauce

Prep: 10 minutes | Cook: 15 minutes | Serves:4

Ingredients:

- 1 cup oat flour (120g)
- 1/2 cup cottage cheese (120g)
- 2 large eggs
- 1/4 cup raisins (40g)
- 1 tsp vanilla extract
- 1/2 tsp baking powder
- 1/4 tsp salt
- 1/2 cup plain yogurt (120g)
- 1 tbsp honey (21g)

Instructions:

1. In a bowl, combine oat flour, baking powder, and salt.
2. In another bowl, whisk cottage cheese, eggs, raisins, and vanilla extract.
3. Mix wet ingredients into dry ingredients until a smooth batter forms.
4. Heat a non-stick pan over medium heat and pour small amounts of batter to make pancakes. Cook until bubbles form, flip and cook the other side.
5. For the yogurt sauce, mix yogurt with honey and serve over pancakes.

Nutritional Facts (Per Serving): Calories: 396 | Protein: 18g | Fat: 13g | Carbs: 58g | Fiber: 5g | Sodium: 770mg | Sugars: 12g

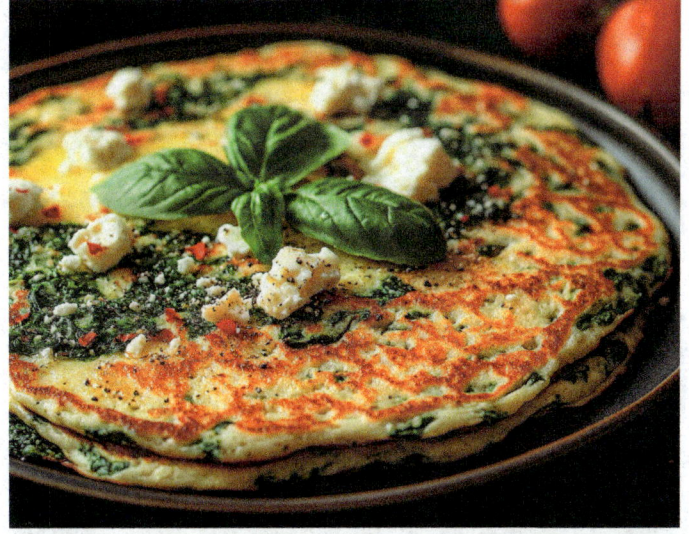

Spinach and Ricotta Pancakes

Prep: 10 minutes | Cook: 15 minutes | Serves:4

Ingredients:

- 1 cup oat flour (120g)
- 1/2 cup low-fat ricotta cheese (60g)
- 1 cup fresh spinach, chopped (40g)
- 2 large eggs
- 1/2 tsp baking powder
- 1/4 tsp salt
- 1/4 tsp black pepper
- 1/3 cup unsweetened oat milk (80ml) (or other gentle milk alternative)
- 1 tbsp olive oil (15ml)

Instructions:

1. In a large bowl, mix oat flour, baking powder, salt, and pepper.
2. In another bowl, whisk eggs, oat milk, and olive oil.
3. Stir in spinach and ricotta cheese.
4. Mix wet ingredients into dry ingredients until well combined.
5. Heat a non-stick skillet over medium heat and pour the batter to form small pancakes. Cook for 3 minutes on each side until golden.
6. Serve warm.

Nutritional Facts (Per Serving): Calories: 378 | Protein: 19g | Fat: 12g | Carbs: 50g | Fiber: 6g | Sodium: 520mg | Sugars: 6g

CHAPTER 4: BREAKFASTS: Easy morning porridges

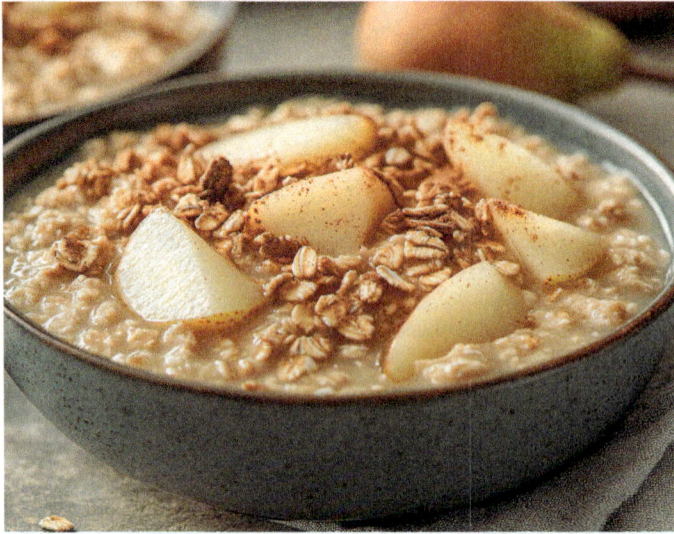

Pear ginger oatmeal

Prep: 5 minutes | Cook: 10 minutes | Serves: 4

Ingredients:

- 1 cup rolled oats (90g)
- 2 cups almond milk (480ml)
- 1 ripe pear, diced (150g)
- 1 tsp grated ginger (2g)
- 1 tbsp honey (21g)
- 1/2 tsp cinnamon
- 1/4 tsp salt (1g)

Instructions:

1. In a saucepan, bring almond milk to a simmer over medium heat.
2. Add oats, diced pear, ginger, cinnamon, and salt. Cook, stirring occasionally, for 5-7 minutes until the oats are soft and the pear is tender.
3. Stir in honey and cook for an additional 2 minutes.
4. Serve warm, garnished with extra pear slices if desired.

Nutritional Facts (Per Serving): Calories: 387 | Protein: 17g | Fat: 14g | Carbs: 58g | Fiber: 7g | Sodium: 760mg | Sugars: 10g

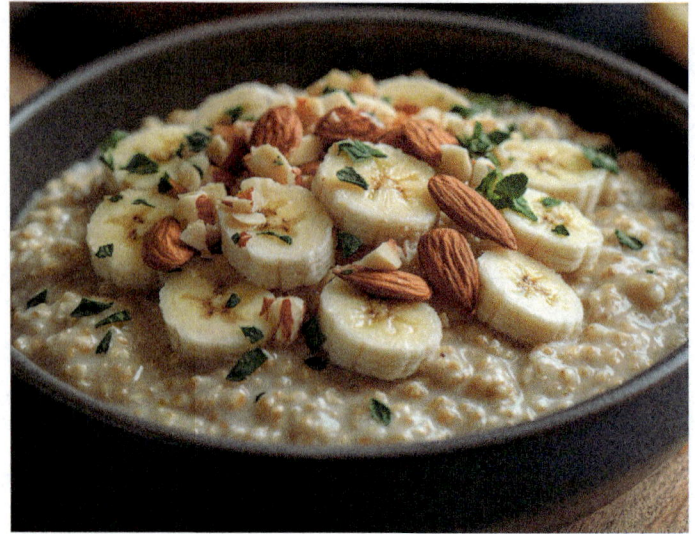

Banana almond buckwheat porridge

Prep: 5 minutes | Cook: 15 minutes | Serves: 4

Ingredients:

- 1 cup buckwheat groats (170g)
- 2 cups water (480ml)
- 1 ripe banana, mashed (120g)
- 1/4 cup almond butter (60g)
- 1 tbsp low carb sweeteners
- 1/2 tsp vanilla extract
- 1/4 cup almond milk (60ml)
- 1/4 tsp salt (1g)

Instructions:

1. Rinse buckwheat groats and add them to a pot with water. Bring to a boil, reduce heat, and simmer for 10-12 minutes until tender.
2. Stir in mashed banana, almond butter, sweetener, vanilla extract, almond milk, and salt.
3. Cook for another 2-3 minutes until creamy.
4. Serve with a drizzle of almond milk and sliced almonds if desired.

Nutritional Facts (Per Serving): Calories: 397 | Protein: 19g | Fat: 15g | Carbs: 56g | Fiber: 6g | Sodium: 750mg | Sugars: 9g

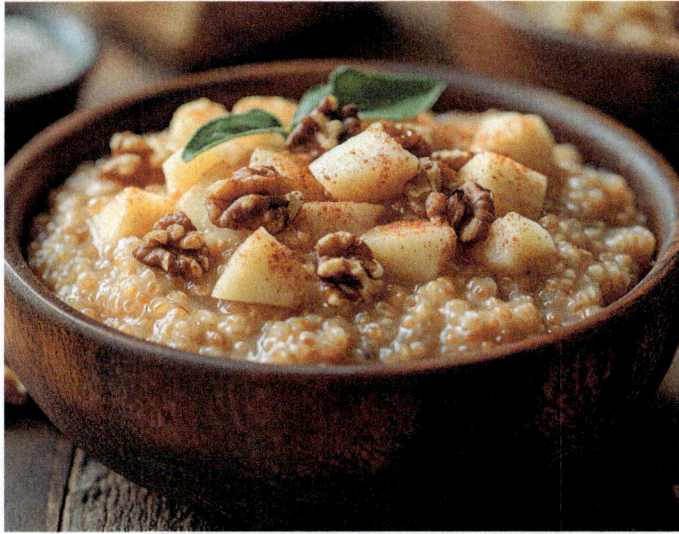

Apple walnut amaranth porridge

Prep: 5 minutes | Cook: 20 minutes | Serves: 4

Ingredients:

- 1 cup amaranth (190g)
- 2 cups water (480ml)
- 1 apple, diced (150g)
- 1/4 cup chopped walnuts (30g)
- 1 tbsp honey (21g)
- 1/2 tsp cinnamon
- 1/4 tsp salt (1g)

Instructions:

1. In a saucepan, bring water to a boil, then add amaranth and reduce to a simmer. Cook for 15-20 minutes until the grains are tender.
2. Stir in diced apple, walnuts, honey, cinnamon, and salt. Cook for another 3-5 minutes until the apple softens.
3. Serve warm with extra walnuts for garnish if desired.

Nutritional Facts (Per Serving): Calories: 387 | Protein: 18g | Fat: 14g | Carbs: 57g | Fiber: 6g | Sodium: 760mg | Sugars: 8g

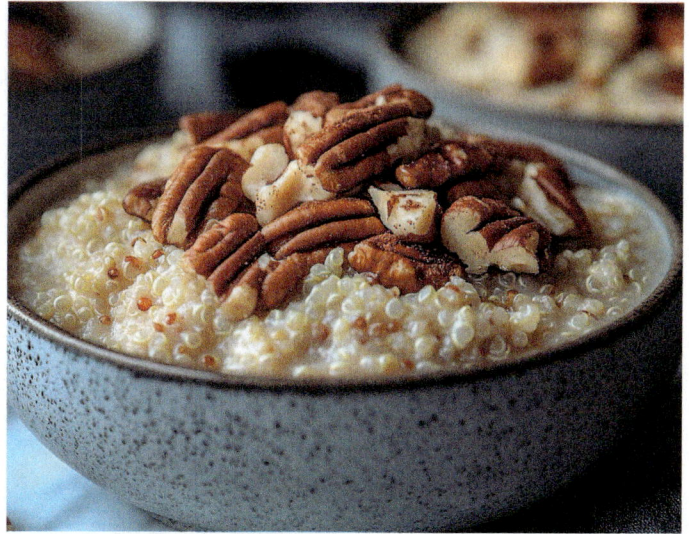

Maple pecan quinoa porridge

Prep: 5 minutes | Cook: 15 minutes | Serves: 4

Ingredients:

- 1 cup quinoa (170g)
- 2 cups almond milk (480ml)
- 2 tbsp maple syrup (42g)
- 1/4 cup pecans, chopped (30g)
- 1/2 tsp cinnamon
- 1/4 tsp salt (1g)

Instructions:

1. Rinse quinoa and add to a pot with almond milk. Bring to a boil, then simmer for 12-15 minutes until quinoa is tender and the liquid is absorbed.
2. Stir in maple syrup, pecans, cinnamon, and salt.
3. Serve warm, topped with extra pecans if desired.

Nutritional Facts (Per Serving): Calories: 396 | Protein: 16g | Fat: 14g | Carbs: 58g | Fiber: 6g | Sodium: 760mg | Sugars: 10

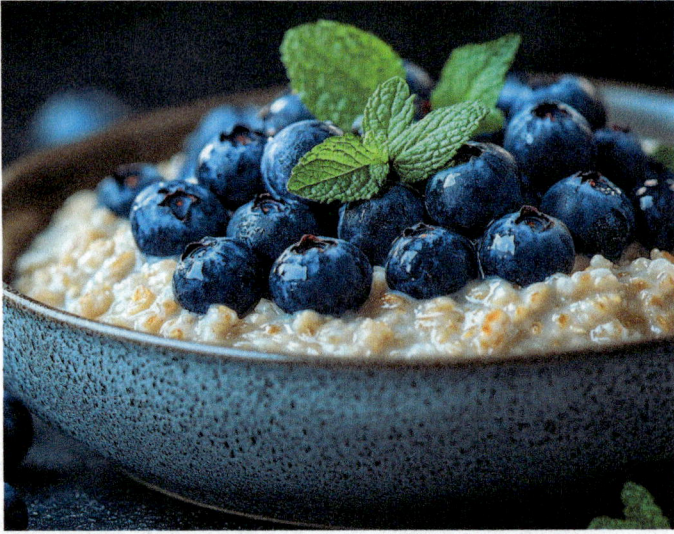

Blueberries vanilla millet porridge

Prep: 5 minutes | Cook: 15 minutes | Serves: 4

Ingredients:

- 1 cup millet (200g)
- 2 cups almond milk (480ml)
- 1 cup fresh blueberries (150g)
- 1 tsp vanilla extract
- 1 tbsp low carb sweeteners
- 1/4 tsp salt (1g)

Instructions:

1. Rinse millet and add to a pot with almond milk. Bring to a boil, then simmer for 15 minutes until millet is tender and most liquid is absorbed.
2. Stir in blueberries, vanilla extract, sweetener, and salt. Cook for another 2 minutes.
3. Serve warm, with extra blueberries if desired.

Nutritional Facts (Per Serving): Calories: 387 | Protein: 17g | Fat: 13g | Carbs: 60g | Fiber: 5g | Sodium: 770mg | Sugars: 8g

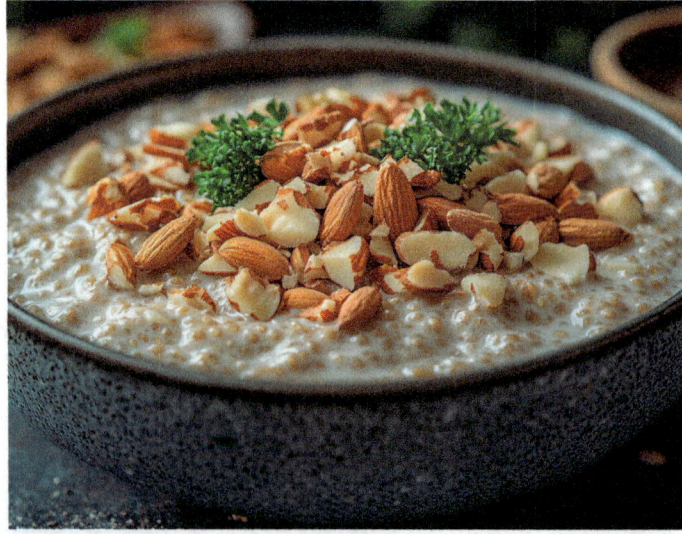

Vanilla chia and flax porridge

Prep: 5 minutes | Cook: 10 minutes | Serves: 4

Ingredients:

- 1/4 cup chia seeds (40g)
- 1/4 cup ground flaxseed (40g)
- 2 cups almond milk (480ml)
- 1 tsp vanilla extract
- 1 tbsp low carb sweeteners
- 1/4 cup chopped almonds (30g)
- 1/4 tsp salt (1g)

Instructions:

1. In a saucepan, combine chia seeds, ground flaxseed, and almond milk. Let sit for 5 minutes to thicken.
2. Stir in vanilla extract, sweetener, almonds, and salt. Heat over low for 5 minutes, stirring occasionally.
3. Serve warm, with additional almonds for garnish.

Nutritional Facts (Per Serving): Calories: 369 | Protein: 18g | Fat: 15g | Carbs: 55g | Fiber: 9g | Sodium: 760mg | Sugars: 7g

CHAPTER 5: BREAKFASTS: Eggs and breakfast proteins

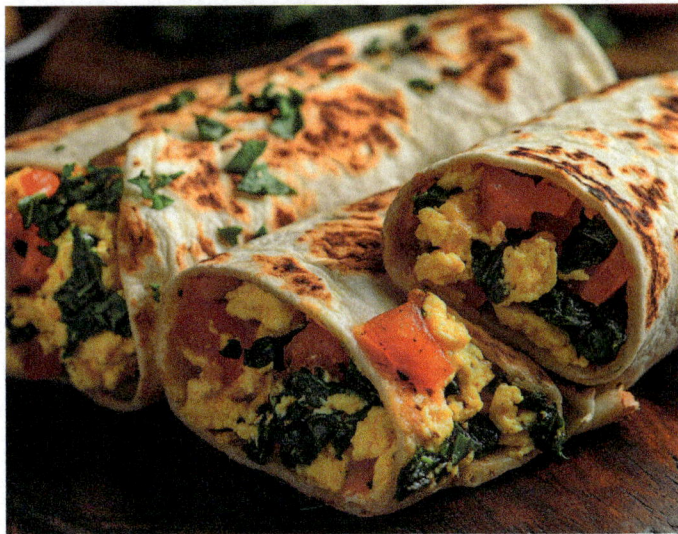

Egg white and vegetable wrap

Prep: 5 minutes | Cook: 10 minutes | Serves: 4

Ingredients:

- 1 cup egg whites (240ml)
- 1/2 cup bell peppers, diced (75g)
- 1/2 cup spinach, chopped (30g)
- 1/4 cup onion, diced (30g)
- 1/4 tsp black pepper
- 1/4 tsp salt
- 4 whole wheat tortillas (120g)
- 1 tbsp olive oil (15ml)

Instructions:

1. Heat olive oil in a non-stick pan over medium heat. Add onions, bell peppers, and spinach, sauté for 3-4 minutes.
2. Pour in the egg whites, season with salt and pepper, and scramble until cooked through.
3. Place the egg white mixture into whole wheat tortillas and wrap.
4. Serve warm.

Nutritional Facts (Per Serving): Calories: 397 | Protein: 20g | Fat: 13g | Carbs: 56g | Fiber: 6g | Sodium: 780mg | Sugars: 7g

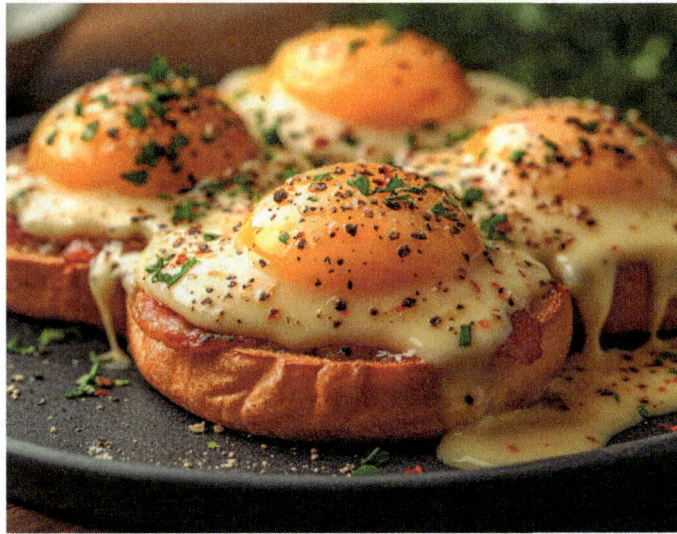

Eggs Benedict

Prep: 10 minutes | Cook: 15 minutes | Serves:4

Ingredients:

- 4 whole wheat English muffins, halved (200g)
- 4 large eggs
- 4 slices turkey bacon (120g)
- 1 tbsp white vinegar (15ml)
- 1/4 cup Greek yogurt (60g)
- 1 tbsp lemon juice (15ml)
- 1/2 tsp Dijon mustard
- 1 tbsp olive oil (15ml)
- 1/4 tsp black pepper
- 1/4 tsp salt (1g)

Instructions:

1. Toast the English muffin halves and cook the turkey bacon until crispy.
2. Poach the eggs: In a pot, bring water with vinegar to a simmer, gently add the eggs, and cook for 3-4 minutes.
3. For the sauce, whisk yogurt, lemon juice, Dijon mustard, olive oil, salt, and pepper in a small bowl.
4. Assemble: Place turkey bacon on the toasted muffins, top with a poached egg, and drizzle with yogurt sauce.

Nutritional Facts (Per Serving): Calories: 386 | Protein: 22g | Fat: 13g | Carbs: 58g | Fiber: 7g | Sodium: 780mg | Sugars: 9g

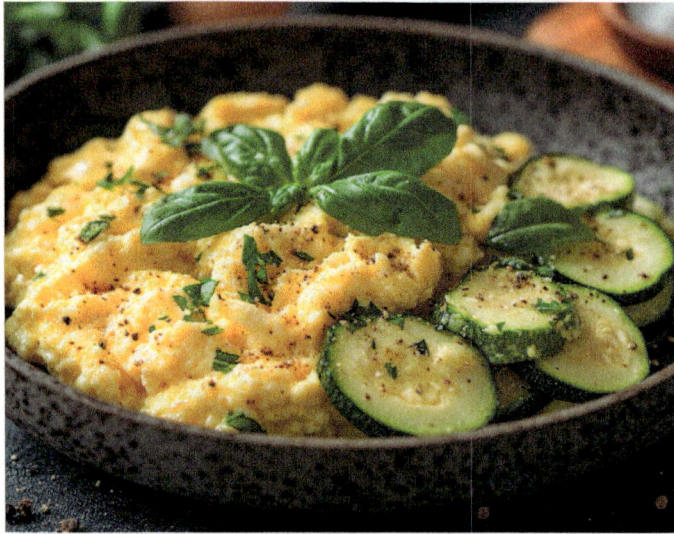

Scrambled eggs with zucchini

Prep: 5 minutes | Cook: 10 minutes | Serves: 4

Ingredients:

- 6 large eggs
- 1 cup zucchini, diced (120g)
- 1/4 cup onion, diced (30g)
- 1 tbsp olive oil (15ml)
- 1/4 tsp black pepper
- 1/4 tsp salt (1g)

Instructions:

1. Heat olive oil in a pan over medium heat, add zucchini and onion, and sauté for 5 minutes until softened.
2. In a bowl, whisk eggs with salt and pepper. Pour the eggs into the pan with zucchini and scramble gently until cooked.
3. Serve warm.

Nutritional Facts (Per Serving): Calories: 394 | Protein: 18g | Fat: 14g | Carbs: 55g | Fiber: 6g | Sodium: 770mg | Sugars: 7g

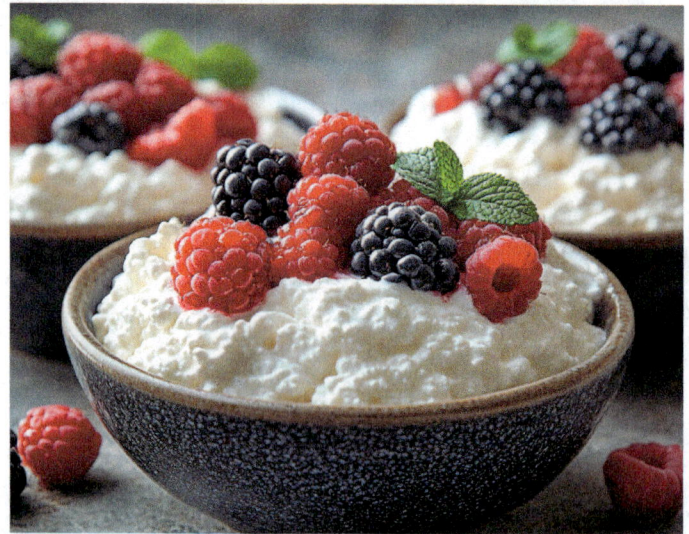

Cottage cheese with seasonal berries and sour cream sauce

Prep: 5 minutes | Cook: 0 minutes | Serves: 4

Ingredients:

- 1 cup cottage cheese (240g)
- 1 cup mixed seasonal berries (150g)
- 1/2 cup sour cream (120g)
- 1 tbsp honey (21g)
- 1 tsp vanilla extract

Instructions:

1. Divide cottage cheese evenly between 4 bowls.
2. Top each serving with mixed seasonal berries.
3. In a small bowl, whisk sour cream, honey, and vanilla extract to create the sauce.
4. Drizzle the sour cream sauce over the cottage cheese and berries.
5. Serve immediately.

Nutritional Facts (Per Serving): Calories: 376 | Protein: 18g | Fat: 14g | Carbs: 56g | Fiber: 6g | Sodium: 760mg | Sugars: 12g

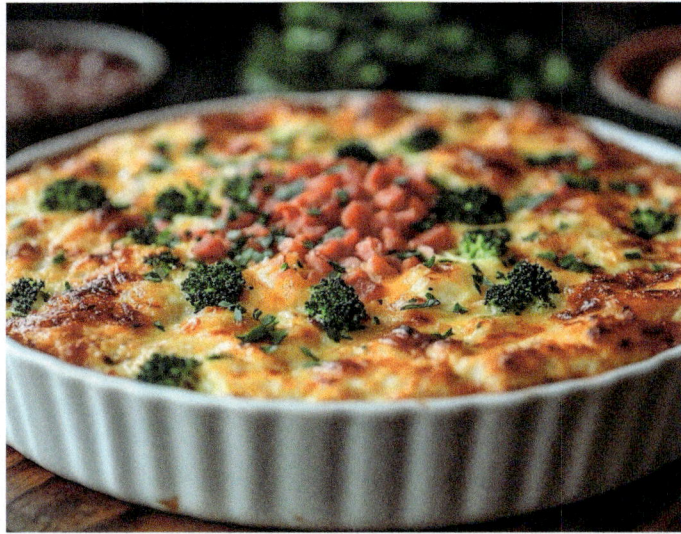

Egg casserole with chicken and broccoli

Prep: 10 minutes | Cook: 30 minutes | Serves:4

Ingredients:

- 6 large eggs
- 1 cup cooked chicken, diced (150g)
- 1 cup broccoli florets, steamed (90g)
- 1/2 cup low-fat cheddar cheese, shredded (60g)
- 1/4 cup almond milk (60ml)
- 1/2 tsp salt (1g)
- 1/4 tsp black pepper

Instructions:

1. Preheat oven to 350°F (175°C) and grease a baking dish.
2. In a bowl, whisk eggs, almond milk, salt, and pepper.
3. Spread diced chicken and steamed broccoli evenly in the baking dish.
4. Pour the egg mixture over the chicken and broccoli and sprinkle shredded cheddar cheese on top.
5. Bake for 30 minutes or until the eggs are set and the top is golden brown.
6. Let cool slightly before serving.

Nutritional Facts (Per Serving): Calories: 396 | Protein: 22g | Fat: 14g | Carbs: 58g | Fiber: 5g | Sodium: 770mg | Sugars: 9g

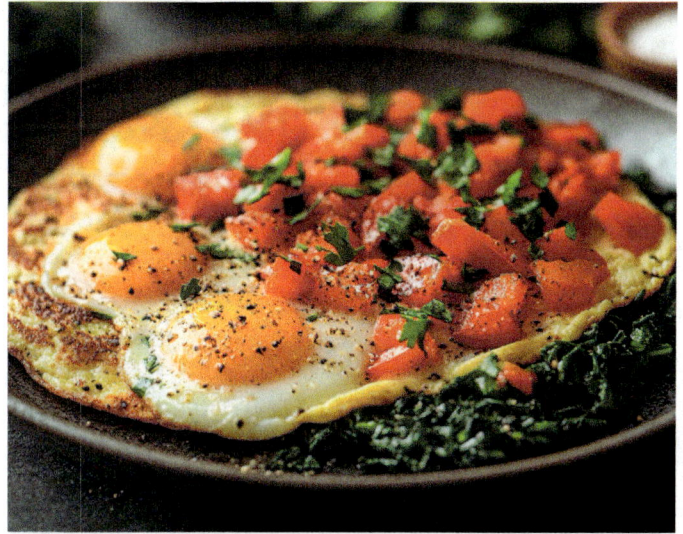

Thin egg pancakes with vegetable filling

Prep: 10 minutes | Cook: 15 minutes | Serves:4

Ingredients:

- 4 large eggs
- 1/4 cup almond milk (60ml)
- 1 tbsp olive oil (15ml)
- 1/4 tsp salt
- 1/4 tsp black pepper
- 1 cup bell peppers, diced (150g)
- 1/2 cup spinach, chopped (30g)
- 1/4 cup onion, diced (30g)

Instructions:

1. In a bowl, whisk eggs, almond milk, salt, and pepper.
2. Heat a non-stick skillet over medium heat and add olive oil.
3. Pour a thin layer of the egg mixture into the skillet and cook for 2-3 minutes until set, then flip and cook the other side. Repeat with the remaining mixture.
4. In a separate pan, sauté bell peppers, spinach, and onion for 5 minutes until soft.
5. Fill the egg pancakes with the sautéed vegetables and fold.
6. Serve warm.

Nutritional Facts (Per Serving): Calories: 375 | Protein: 19g | Fat: 13g | Carbs: 55g | Fiber: 6g | Sodium: 780mg | Sugars: 8g

CHAPTER 6: BREAKFASTS: Cooking with pleasure on weekends

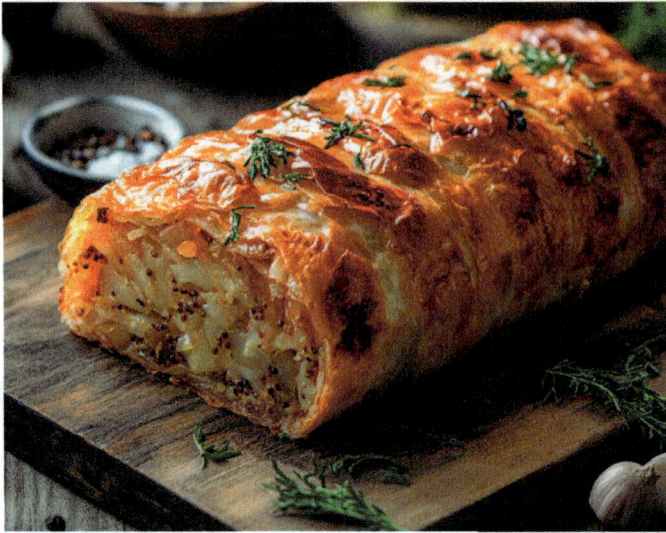

Cabbage strudel

Prep: 15 minutes | Cook: 25 minutes | Serves:4

Ingredients:

- 2 cups shredded cabbage (180g)
- 1 small onion, diced (50g)
- 1 tbsp olive oil (15ml)
- 1/2 tsp caraway seeds
- 6 sheets whole wheat phyllo dough (180g)
- 1 tbsp low carb sweeteners
- 1/4 tsp salt (1g)
- 1/4 tsp black pepper
- 1 tbsp olive oil for brushing (15ml)

Instructions:

1. Preheat oven to 375°F (190°C).
2. Heat olive oil in a pan, sauté onion and cabbage with caraway seeds until softened. Season with salt and pepper.
3. Lay out phyllo dough sheets, brushing each layer lightly with olive oil.
4. Spread the cabbage mixture on one edge of the dough, roll it up to form a strudel.
5. Bake for 25 minutes or until golden and crisp. Let cool slightly before slicing.

Nutritional Facts (Per Serving): Calories: 407 | Protein: 16g | Fat: 14g | Carbs: 56g | Fiber: 6g | Sodium: 780mg | Sugars: 8g

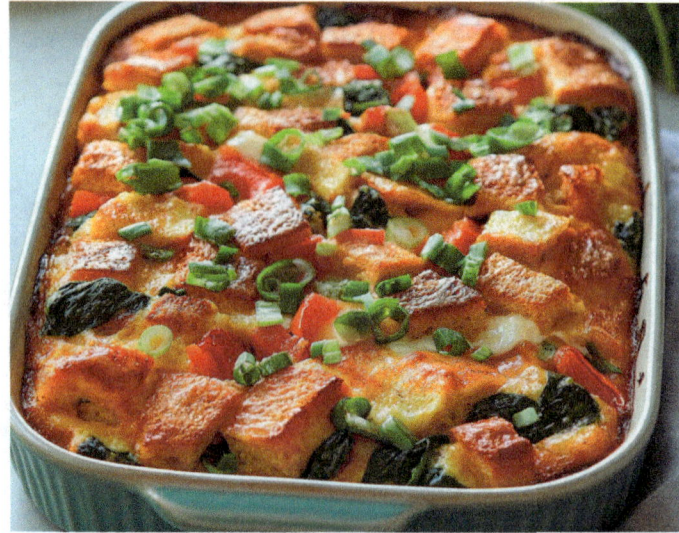

Vegetable and cheese strata

Prep: 10 minutes | Cook: 30 minutes | Serves:4

Ingredients:

- 4 slices whole wheat bread, cubed (120g)
- 1 cup spinach, chopped (40g)
- 1/2 cup bell peppers, diced (75g)
- 1/2 cup shredded low-fat cheddar cheese (60g)
- 4 large eggs
- 1/2 cup almond milk (120ml)
- 1/4 tsp salt
- 1/4 tsp black pepper

Instructions:

1. Preheat oven to 350°F (175°C) and grease a baking dish.
2. In a bowl, whisk eggs, almond milk, salt, and pepper.
3. Layer cubed bread, spinach, bell peppers, and cheese in the baking dish. Pour the egg mixture over the layers.
4. Bake for 30 minutes or until golden brown and set.
5. Cool for a few minutes before serving.

Nutritional Facts (Per Serving): Calories: 395 | Protein: 19g | Fat: 14g | Carbs: 58g | Fiber: 5g | Sodium: 770mg | Sugars: 9g

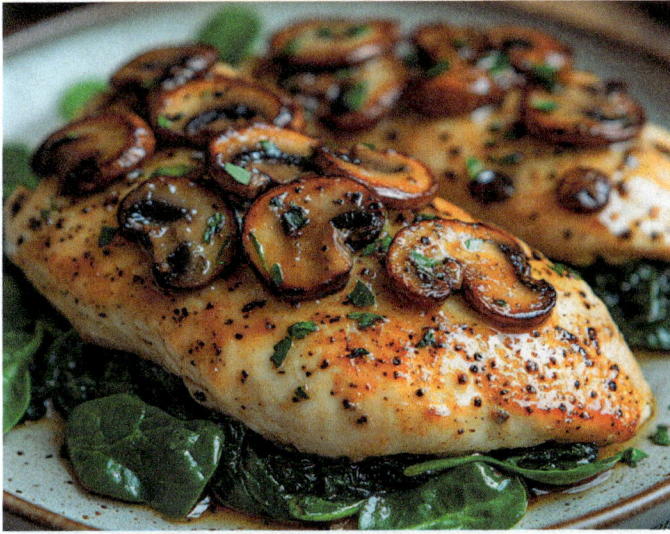

Spinach and mushroom stuffed chicken breast

Prep: 10 minutes | Cook: 25 minutes | Serves:4

Ingredients:

- 4 chicken breasts, boneless (500g)
- 1 cup spinach, chopped (40g)
- 1/2 cup mushrooms, sliced (90g)
- 1/4 cup low-fat cream cheese (60g)
- 1 tbsp olive oil (15ml)
- 1/4 tsp salt (1g)
- 1/4 tsp black pepper
- 1/2 tsp garlic powder

Instructions:

1. Preheat oven to 375°F (190°C). Cut a pocket into each chicken breast.
2. Sauté spinach and mushrooms in olive oil until softened, season with salt, pepper, and garlic powder.
3. Mix the sautéed vegetables with cream cheese and stuff each chicken breast.
4. Place stuffed chicken breasts in a baking dish and bake for 25 minutes until cooked through.
5. Let cool for a few minutes before slicing.

Nutritional Facts (Per Serving): Calories: 387 | Protein: 25g | Fat: 13g | Carbs: 55g | Fiber: 6g | Sodium: 780mg | Sugars: 8g

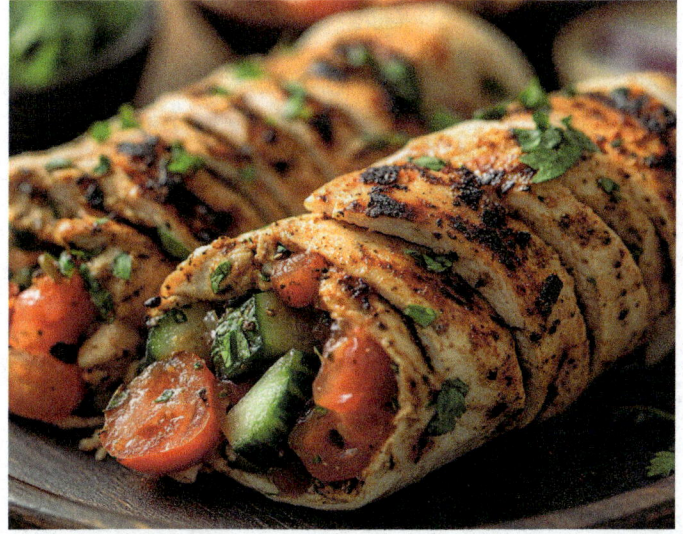

Mediterranean chicken wrap

Prep: 10 minutes | Cook: 15 minutes | Serves:4

Ingredients:

- 2 chicken breasts, sliced (300g)
- 1 tbsp olive oil (15ml)
- 1 tsp dried oregano
- 1/2 tsp ground cumin
- 1/4 tsp salt
- 1/4 tsp black pepper
- 1 cup cucumber, diced (150g)
- 1/2 cup cherry tomatoes, halved (75g)
- 1/4 cup red onion, sliced (30g)
- 4 whole wheat tortillas (120g)
- 1/4 cup hummus (60g)

Instructions:

1. In a bowl, mix olive oil, oregano, cumin, salt, and pepper. Coat the chicken slices with the seasoning mix.
2. Cook the chicken in a pan over medium heat for 10-12 minutes until fully cooked.
3. In each tortilla, spread hummus, then add chicken, cucumber, tomatoes, and red onion.
4. Wrap tightly and serve.

Nutritional Facts (Per Serving): Calories: 395 | Protein: 24g | Fat: 14g | Carbs: 55g | Fiber: 6g | Sodium: 780mg | Sugars: 7g

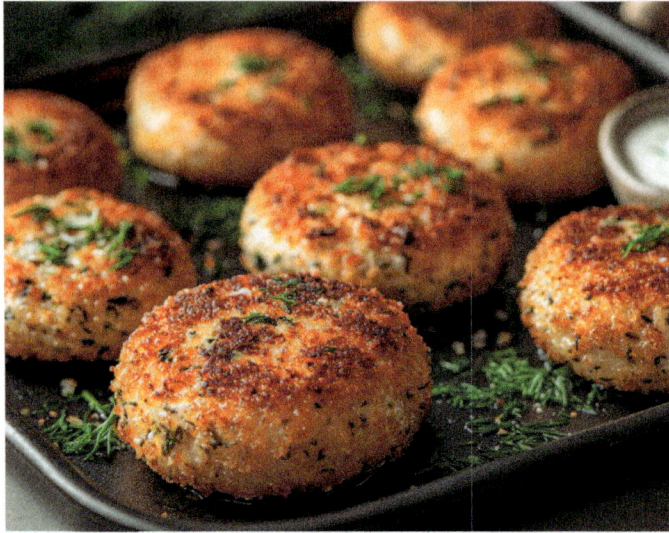

Baked mushroom fritters with sour cream sauce

Prep: 10 minutes | Cook: 20 minutes | Serves:4

Ingredients:

- 2 cups mushrooms, finely chopped (180g)
- 1/4 cup whole wheat breadcrumbs (30g)
- 1 large egg
- 1/4 cup low-fat sour cream (60g)
- 1 tbsp olive oil (15ml)
- 1/2 tsp garlic powder
- 1/4 tsp salt
- 1/4 tsp black pepper

For the sauce:
- 1/2 cup low-fat sour cream (120g)
- 1 tbsp lemon juice (15ml)
- 1/4 tsp dill, chopped

Instructions:

1. Preheat oven to 375°F (190°C) and line a baking sheet with parchment paper.
2. In a bowl, mix chopped mushrooms, breadcrumbs, egg, garlic powder, salt, and pepper.
3. Form small patties and place them on the baking sheet. Brush each with olive oil.
4. Bake for 15-20 minutes until golden.
5. For the sauce, whisk sour cream, lemon juice, and dill together.
6. Serve the fritters with sour cream sauce.

Nutritional Facts (Per Serving): Calories: 386 | Protein: 18g | Fat: 13g | Carbs: 55g | Fiber: 5g | Sodium: 770mg | Sugars: 8g

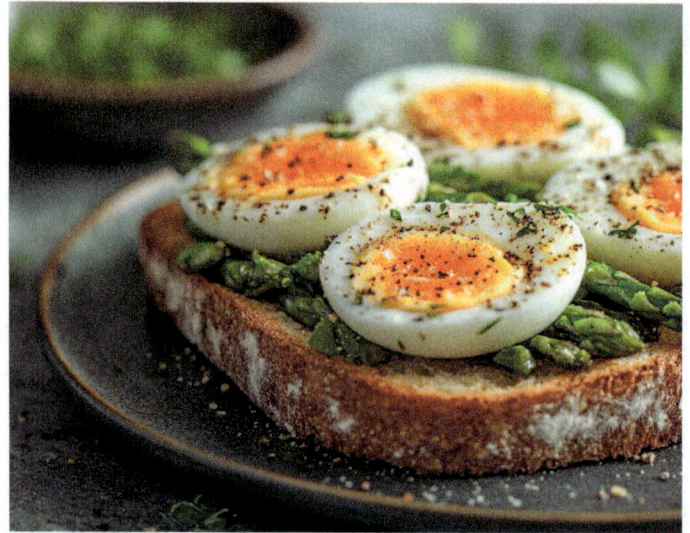

Bruschetta with boiled eggs, soft cheese, and asparagus

Prep: 10 minutes | Cook: 15 minutes | Serves:4

Ingredients:

- 4 slices whole wheat bread (120g)
- 4 boiled eggs, sliced
- 1/2 cup soft goat cheese (120g)
- 8 asparagus spears, steamed (120g)
- 1 tbsp olive oil (15ml)
- 1/4 tsp black pepper
- 1/4 tsp salt (1g)

Instructions:

1. Toast the whole wheat bread slices until golden.
2. Spread goat cheese evenly over each slice.
3. Top with sliced boiled eggs and steamed asparagus spears.
4. Drizzle with olive oil and season with salt and pepper.
5. Serve warm.

Nutritional Facts (Per Serving): Calories: 379 | Protein: 19g | Fat: 14g | Carbs: 55g | Fiber: 6g | Sodium: 780mg | Sugars: 7g

CHAPTER 7: BREAKFASTS: Low-Acid, delicate smoothies, shakes and juices

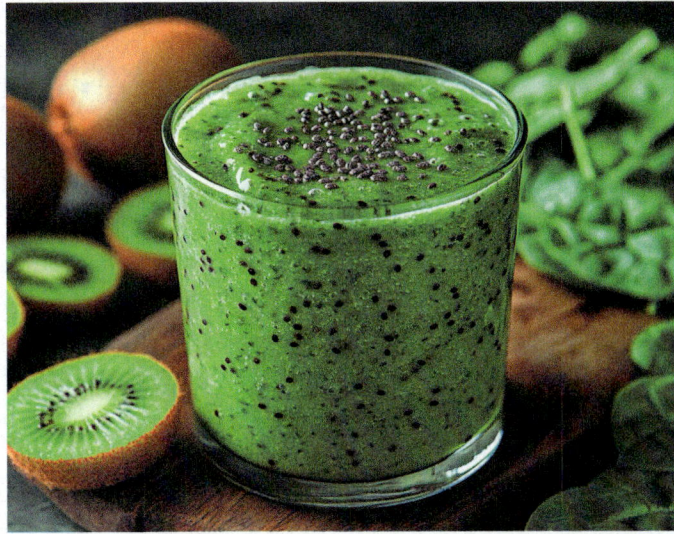

Kiwi and spinach smoothie

Prep: 5 minutes | Cook: 0 minutes | Serves: 2

Ingredients:

- 2 kiwis, peeled and chopped (200g)
- 1 cup fresh spinach (30g)
- 1 cup coconut water (240ml)
- 1 tbsp low carb sweeteners

Instructions:

1. Add kiwis, spinach, coconut water, and sweetener to a blender.
2. Blend until smooth and serve immediately.

Nutritional Facts (Per Serving): Calories: 360 | Protein: 18g | Fat: 14g | Carbs: 58g | Fiber: 7g | Sodium: 780mg | Sugars: 12g

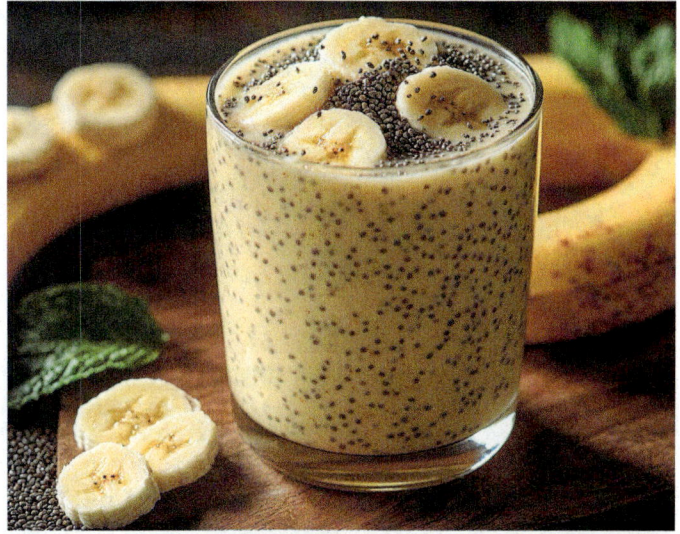

Banana and chia seed shake

Prep: 5 minutes | Cook: 0 minutes | Serves: 2

Ingredients:

- 2 ripe bananas (240g)
- 2 tbsp chia seeds (30g)
- 2 cups almond milk (480ml)
- 1 tbsp low carb sweeteners

Instructions:

1. Add bananas, chia seeds, almond milk, and sweetener to a blender.
2. Blend until smooth and serve chilled.

Nutritional Facts (Per Serving): Calories: 387 | Protein: 19g | Fat: 13g | Carbs: 60g | Fiber: 8g | Sodium: 770mg | Sugars: 10g

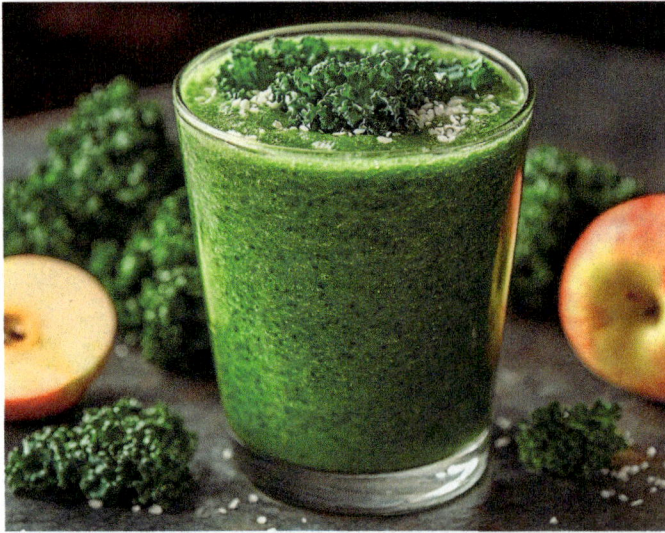

Apple and kale smoothie

Prep: 5 minutes | Cook: 0 minutes | Serves: 2

Ingredients:

- 1 large apple, cored and chopped (180g)
- 1 cup fresh kale (30g)
- 1 cup coconut water (240ml)
- 1 tbsp low carb sweeteners

Instructions:

1. Add apple, kale, coconut water, and sweetener to a blender.
2. Blend until smooth and serve immediately.

Nutritional Facts (Per Serving): Calories: 393 | Protein: 17g | Fat: 14g | Carbs: 57g | Fiber: 6g | Sodium: 760mg | Sugars: 11g

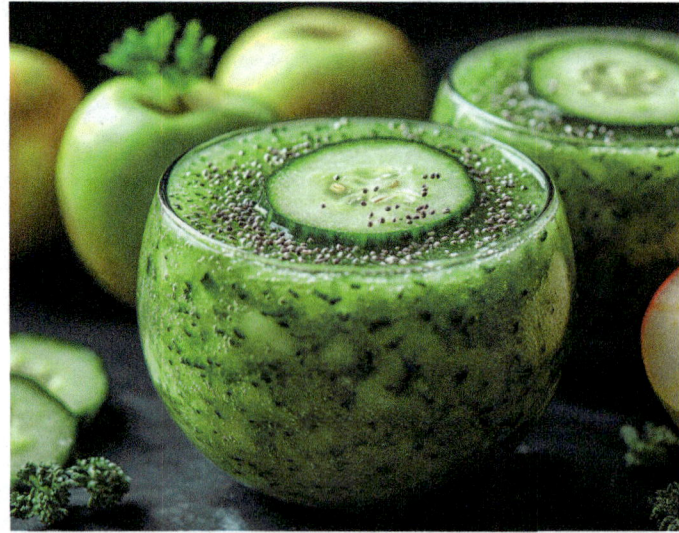

Cucumber and apple smoothie

Prep: 5 minutes | Cook: 0 minutes | Serves: 2

Ingredients:

- 1 large cucumber, peeled and chopped (200g)
- 1 large apple, cored and chopped (180g)
- 1 cup coconut water (240ml)
- 1 tbsp low carb sweeteners

Instructions:

1. Add cucumber, apple, coconut water, and sweetener to a blender.
2. Blend until smooth and serve immediately.

Nutritional Facts (Per Serving): Calories: 386 | Protein: 18g | Fat: 14g | Carbs: 58g | Fiber: 6g | Sodium: 770mg | Sugars: 10g

CHAPTER 8: LUNCHES: Soothing soups and wholesome stews

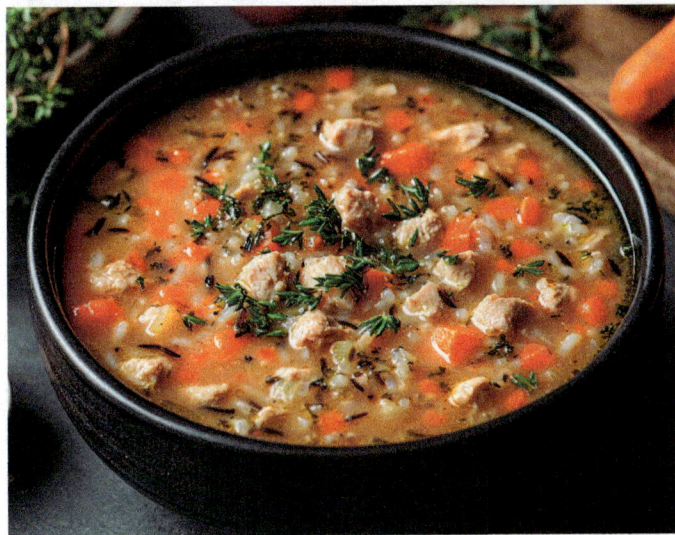

Turkey and wild rice soup

Prep: 10 minutes | Cook: 30 minutes | Serves:4

Ingredients:

- 1 lb ground turkey (450g)
- 1/2 cup wild rice (90g)
- 2 carrots, diced (120g)
- 2 celery stalks, diced (100g)
- 4 cups turkey broth (960ml)
- 1 tsp dried thyme
- 1/2 tsp black pepper
- 1/2 tsp salt
- 1 tbsp olive oil (15ml)

Instructions:

1. Heat olive oil in a large pot over medium heat. Add ground turkey and cook until browned.
2. Add diced carrots and celery, sauté for 5 minutes.
3. Stir in wild rice, turkey broth, thyme, pepper, and salt. Bring to a boil.
4. Reduce heat, cover, and simmer for 25-30 minutes until rice is tender.
5. Serve warm.

Nutritional Facts (Per Serving): Calories: 489 | Protein: 17g | Fat: 11g | Carbs: 45g | Fiber: 7g | Sodium: 530mg | Sugars: 6g

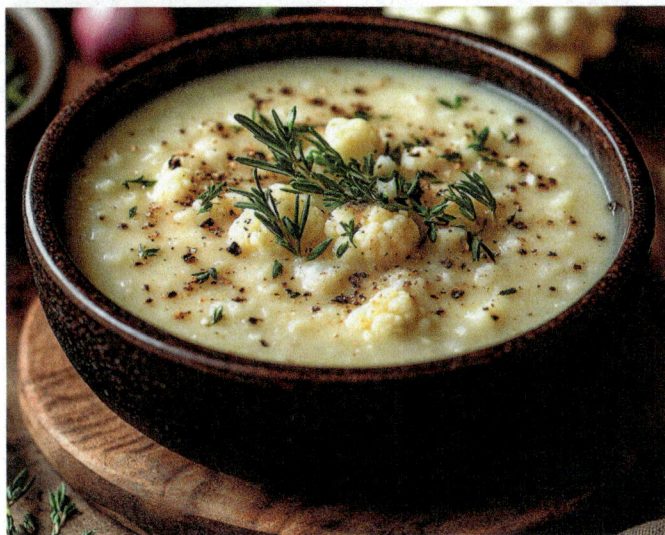

Creamy cauliflower soup

Prep: 10 minutes | Cook: 20 minutes | Serves:4

Ingredients:

- 1 large head cauliflower, chopped (600g)
- 2 cups almond milk (480ml)
- 1 onion, diced (120g)
- 3 cloves garlic, minced (9g)
- 1 tbsp olive oil (15ml)
- 1/2 tsp salt
- 1/4 tsp black pepper
- 1/4 tsp ground nutmeg

Instructions:

1. Heat olive oil in a large pot over medium heat. Add onion and garlic, sauté for 5 minutes until softened.
2. Add cauliflower and almond milk. Bring to a boil, then reduce heat and simmer for 15 minutes until the cauliflower is tender.
3. Blend the soup until smooth using a blender or immersion blender. Season with salt, pepper, and nutmeg.
4. Serve warm.

Nutritional Facts (Per Serving): Calories: 498 | Protein: 16g | Fat: 12g | Carbs: 46g | Fiber: 7g | Sodium: 530mg | Sugars: 8g

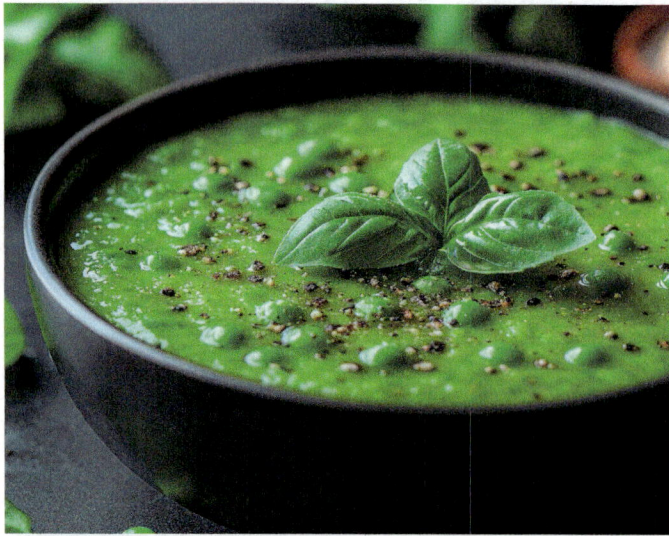

Green pea and basil soup

Prep: 10 minutes | Cook: 15 minutes | Serves:4

Ingredients:

- 4 cups green peas (600g)
- 1 cup fresh basil leaves (25g)
- 1 onion, diced (120g)
- 4 cups vegetable broth (960ml)
- 1 tbsp olive oil (15ml)
- 1/2 tsp salt
- 1/4 tsp black pepper

Instructions:

1. Heat olive oil in a pot over medium heat. Add onion and sauté for 5 minutes until softened.
2. Add peas, broth, salt, and pepper. Bring to a boil, then reduce heat and simmer for 10 minutes.
3. Stir in fresh basil, then blend the soup until smooth.
4. Serve warm.

Nutritional Facts (Per Serving): Calories: 487 | Protein: 14g | Fat: 11g | Carbs: 45g | Fiber: 8g | Sodium: 540mg | Sugars: 6g

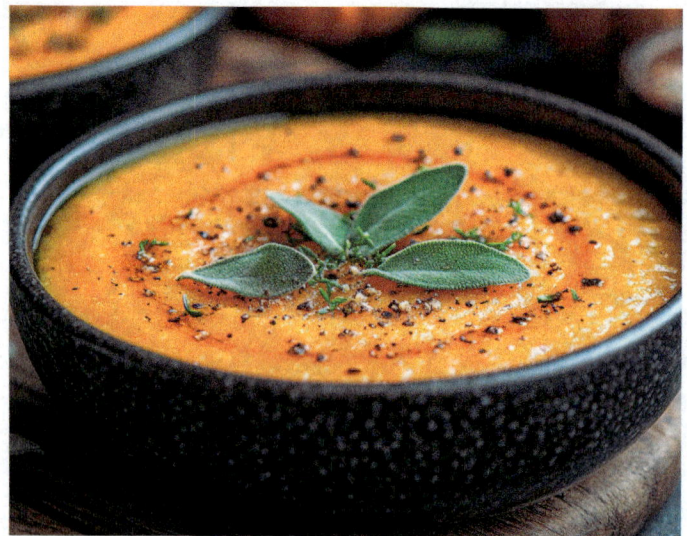

Pumpkin and sage mashed soup

Prep: 10 minutes | Cook: 20 minutes | Serves:4

Ingredients:

- 2 cups pumpkin puree (480g)
- 1 onion, diced (120g)
- 4 cups vegetable broth (960ml)
- 1 tbsp fresh sage, chopped (2g)
- 1 tbsp olive oil (15ml)
- 1/2 tsp salt
- 1/4 tsp black pepper

Instructions:

1. Heat olive oil in a pot over medium heat. Add onion and sage, sauté for 5 minutes until softened.
2. Stir in pumpkin puree, broth, salt, and pepper. Bring to a boil, then reduce heat and simmer for 15 minutes.
3. Blend the soup until smooth and serve warm.

Nutritional Facts (Per Serving): Calories: 496 | Protein: 13g | Fat: 11g | Carbs: 46g | Fiber: 7g | Sodium: 520mg | Sugars: 7g

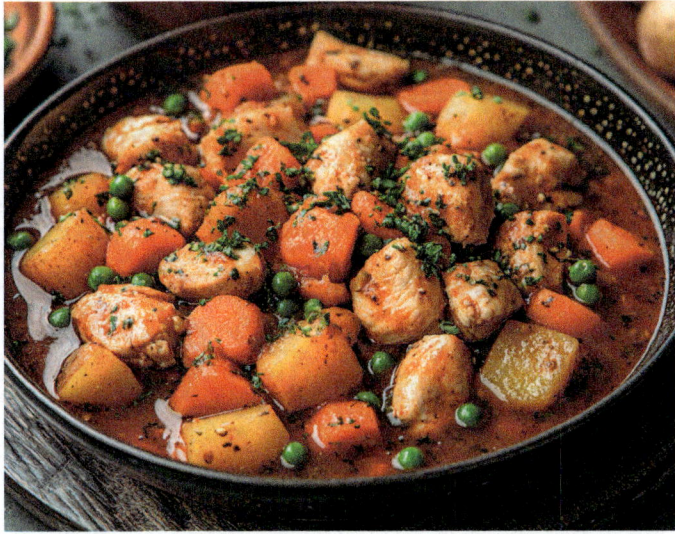

Chicken and vegetable stew

Prep: 15 minutes | Cook: 40 minutes | Serves:4

Ingredients:

- 1 lb chicken breast, diced (450g)
- 2 carrots, diced (120g)
- 2 potatoes, diced (300g)
- 1/2 cup peas (75g)
- 4 cups chicken broth (960ml)
- 1 tbsp olive oil (15ml)
- 1/2 tsp thyme
- 1/4 tsp salt
- 1/4 tsp black pepper

Instructions:

1. Heat olive oil in a large pot over medium heat. Add chicken breast and cook until lightly browned.
2. Add carrots, potatoes, and peas. Stir for 3-4 minutes.
3. Pour in the chicken broth and add thyme, salt, and black pepper. Bring to a boil, then reduce heat to low.
4. Cover and simmer for 30-35 minutes until vegetables are tender and the chicken is fully cooked.
5. Serve warm.

Nutritional Facts (Per Serving): Calories: 486 | Protein: 18g | Fat: 11g | Carbs: 45g | Fiber: 7g | Sodium: 520mg | Sugars: 6g

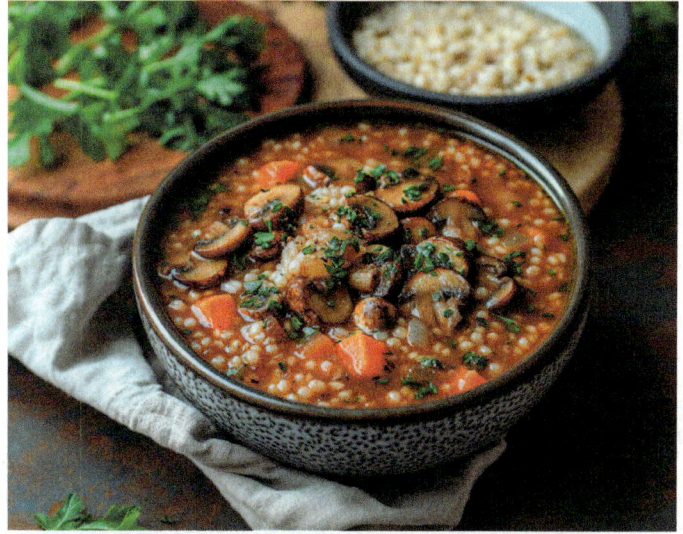

Mushroom barley stew

Prep: 10 minutes | Cook: 45 minutes | Serves:4

Ingredients:

- 2 cups mushrooms, sliced (180g)
- 1/2 cup pearl barley (90g)
- 1 onion, diced (120g)
- 2 carrots, diced (120g)
- 4 cups vegetable broth (960ml)
- 1 tbsp olive oil (15ml)
- 1/2 tsp thyme
- 1/4 tsp salt
- 1/4 tsp black pepper

Instructions:

1. Heat olive oil in a large pot over medium heat. Add onions and carrots, sauté for 5 minutes until softened.
2. Add mushrooms and barley, stirring for 3-4 minutes.
3. Pour in vegetable broth, add thyme, salt, and pepper. Bring to a boil, then reduce heat to low.
4. Cover and simmer for 40-45 minutes until barley is tender.
5. Serve warm.

Nutritional Facts (Per Serving): Calories: 495 | Protein: 13g | Fat: 11g | Carbs: 45g | Fiber: 8g | Sodium: 520mg | Sugars: 6g

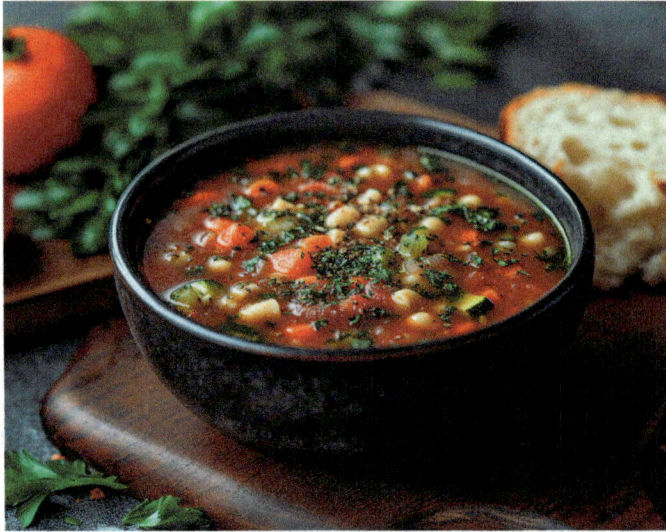

Minestrone soup

Prep: 15 minutes | Cook: 30 minutes | Serves:4

Ingredients:

- 1 cup diced zucchini (150g)
- 1/2 cup diced carrots (75g)
- 1/2 cup diced celery (75g)
- 1 onion, diced (120g)
- 1 can diced tomatoes (400g)
- 1 cup small pasta (100g)
- 4 cups vegetable broth (960ml)
- 1 tbsp olive oil (15ml)
- 1/2 tsp Italian seasoning
- 1/4 tsp salt
- 1/4 tsp black pepper

Instructions:

1. Heat olive oil in a large pot over medium heat. Add onions, carrots, and celery, sauté for 5 minutes until softened.
2. Stir in zucchini, tomatoes, vegetable broth, Italian seasoning, salt, and pepper. Bring to a boil.
3. Add pasta and cook for another 10-12 minutes until pasta is tender.
4. Serve warm.

Nutritional Facts (Per Serving): Calories: 486 | Protein: 14g | Fat: 11g | Carbs: 45g | Fiber: 7g | Sodium: 510mg | Sugars: 7g

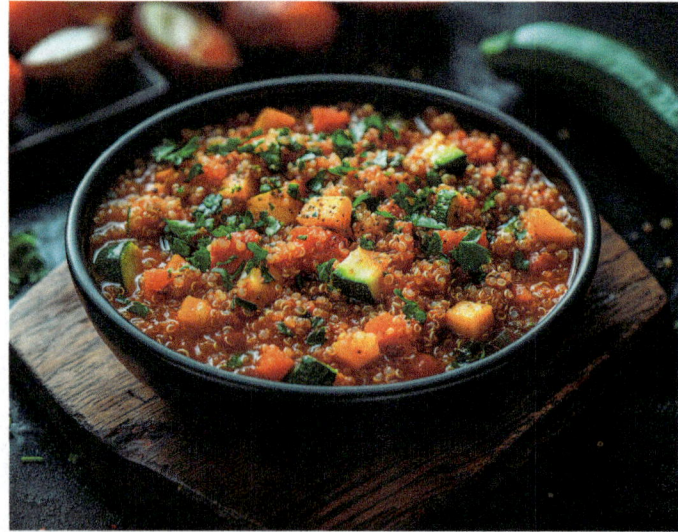

Quinoa and vegetable stew

Prep: 10 minutes | Cook: 25 minutes | Serves:4

Ingredients:

- 1 cup quinoa (170g)
- 1 cup diced zucchini (150g)
- 1/2 cup diced bell peppers (75g)
- 1 cup diced tomatoes (150g)
- 4 cups vegetable broth (960ml)
- 1 tbsp olive oil (15ml)
- 1/2 tsp cumin
- 1/4 tsp salt
- 1/4 tsp black pepper

Instructions:

1. Heat olive oil in a large pot over medium heat. Add quinoa and toast for 2-3 minutes.
2. Add zucchini, bell peppers, tomatoes, vegetable broth, cumin, salt, and pepper. Bring to a boil.
3. Reduce heat, cover, and simmer for 20 minutes until quinoa is tender.
4. Serve warm.

Nutritional Facts (Per Serving): Calories: 498 | Protein: 16g | Fat: 11g | Carbs: 46g | Fiber: 7g | Sodium: 520mg | Sugars: 6g

CHAPTER 9: LUNCHES: Gentle flavors: Low-Acid pasta and risotto

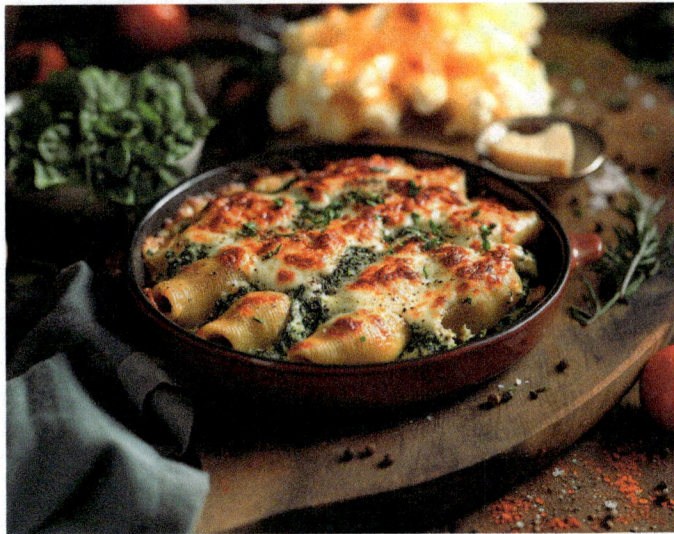

Spinach and ricotta stuffed shells

Prep: 15 minutes | Cook: 25 minutes | Serves:4

Ingredients:

- 12 whole wheat pasta shells (120g)
- 1 cup ricotta cheese (240g)
- 1 cup fresh spinach, chopped (40g)
- 1/4 cup Parmesan cheese, grated (30g)
- 1 egg, beaten
- 1/2 tsp salt
- 1/4 tsp black pepper

Instructions:

1. Preheat the oven to 375°F (190°C). Cook pasta shells according to package instructions.
2. In a bowl, mix ricotta, spinach, Parmesan, egg, salt, and pepper.
3. Stuff each cooked pasta shell with the ricotta mixture and place in a baking dish.
4. Bake for 25 minutes until golden and heated through.
5. Serve warm.

Nutritional Facts (Per Serving): Calories: 487 | Protein: 18g | Fat: 12g | Carbs: 45g | Fiber: 7g | Sodium: 520mg | Sugars: 6g

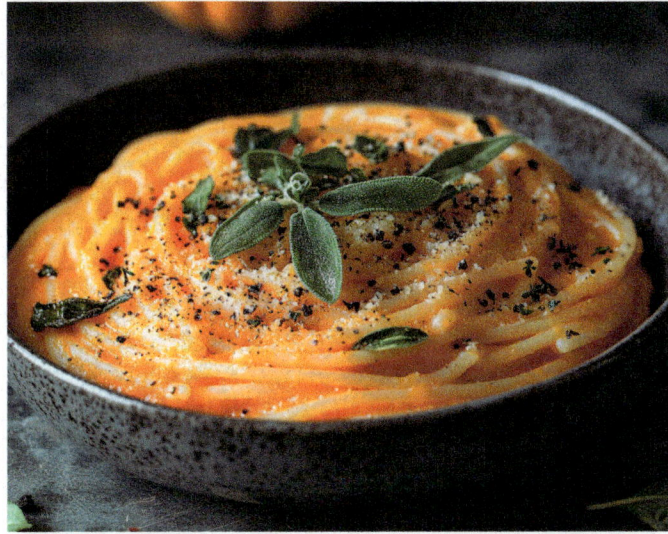

Pumpkin sage pasta

Prep: 10 minutes | Cook: 15 minutes | Serves:4

Ingredients:

- 8 oz whole wheat pasta (225g)
- 1 cup pumpkin puree (240g)
- 1/2 cup almond milk (120ml)
- 1 tbsp fresh sage, chopped (2g)
- 1 tbsp olive oil (15ml)
- 1/4 tsp salt
- 1/4 tsp black pepper

Instructions:

1. Cook the pasta according to package instructions.
2. In a pan, heat olive oil over medium heat. Add pumpkin puree, almond milk, sage, salt, and pepper. Cook for 5 minutes until the sauce thickens.
3. Toss the cooked pasta in the sauce and mix well.
4. Serve warm.

Nutritional Facts (Per Serving): Calories: 496 | Protein: 15g | Fat: 11g | Carbs: 46g | Fiber: 8g | Sodium: 500mg | Sugars: 7g

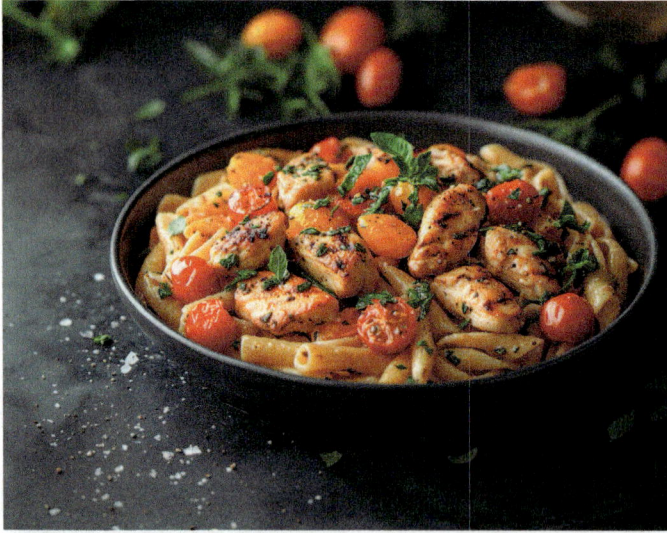

Herb chicken pasta primavera

Prep: 15 minutes | Cook: 20 minutes | Serves:4

Ingredients:

- 8 oz whole wheat pasta (225g)
- 2 chicken breasts, grilled and sliced (300g)
- 1 cup bell peppers, sliced (150g)
- 1/2 cup zucchini, sliced (75g)
- 1/2 cup cherry tomatoes, halved (75g)
- 1 tbsp olive oil (15ml)
- 1 tbsp mixed herbs (oregano, thyme) (2g)
- 1/4 tsp salt
- 1/4 tsp black pepper

Instructions:

1. Cook the pasta according to package instructions.
2. In a pan, heat olive oil over medium heat. Add bell peppers, zucchini, and cherry tomatoes. Sauté for 5-7 minutes until tender.
3. Toss the cooked pasta with the grilled chicken and vegetables. Add mixed herbs, salt, and pepper.
4. Serve warm.

Nutritional Facts (Per Serving): Calories: 487 | Protein: 19g | Fat: 11g | Carbs: 45g | Fiber: 7g | Sodium: 530mg | Sugars: 5g

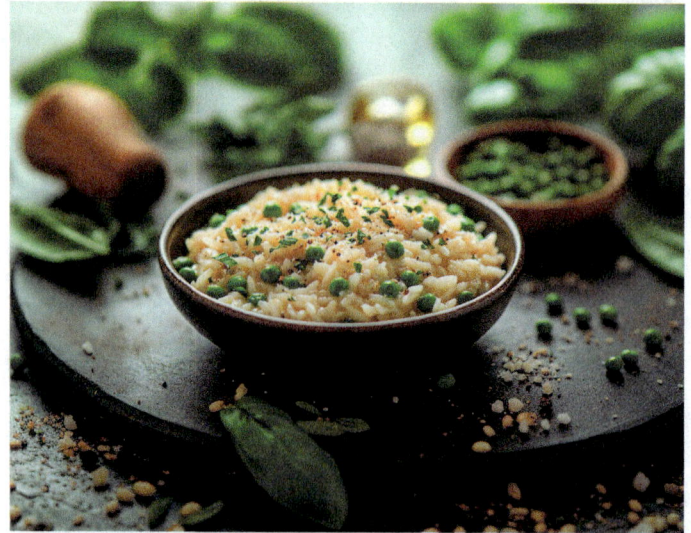

Pea and parmesan risotto

Prep: 10 minutes | Cook: 25 minutes | Serves:4

Ingredients:

- 1 cup brown rice (180g)
- 1 cup green peas (150g)
- 1/2 cup grated Parmesan (50g)
- 4 cups vegetable broth (960ml)
- 1 tbsp olive oil (15ml)
- 1/4 tsp salt
- 1/4 tsp black pepper

Instructions:

1. Heat olive oil in a pan over medium heat. Add rice and stir for 2-3 minutes.
2. Slowly add vegetable broth, one cup at a time, allowing the rice to absorb the liquid before adding more. Stir frequently.
3. When rice is tender (about 20 minutes), stir in green peas, Parmesan, salt, and pepper.
4. Serve warm.

Nutritional Facts (Per Serving): Calories: 479 | Protein: 15g | Fat: 11g | Carbs: 46g | Fiber: 6g | Sodium: 500mg | Sugars: 6g

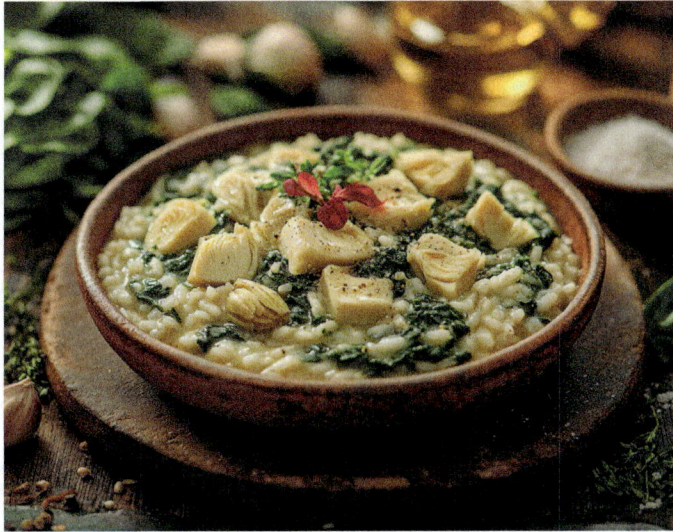

Spinach and artichoke risotto

Prep: 10 minutes | Cook: 25 minutes | Serves:4

Ingredients:

- 1 cup brown rice (180g)
- 1 cup fresh spinach, chopped (30g)
- 1/2 cup artichoke hearts, chopped (100g)
- 1/2 cup light cream (120ml)
- 4 cups vegetable broth (960ml)
- 1 tbsp olive oil (15ml)
- 1/4 tsp salt (1g)
- 1/4 tsp black pepper

Instructions:

1. Heat olive oil in a pan over medium heat. Add rice and cook for 2-3 minutes, stirring.
2. Gradually add vegetable broth, stirring often, until the rice is tender and the broth is absorbed (about 20 minutes).
3. Stir in spinach, artichokes, light cream, salt, and pepper. Cook for an additional 3-4 minutes.
4. Serve warm.

Nutritional Facts (Per Serving): Calories: 493 | Protein: 14g | Fat: 12g | Carbs: 45g | Fiber: 7g | Sodium: 520mg | Sugars: 5g

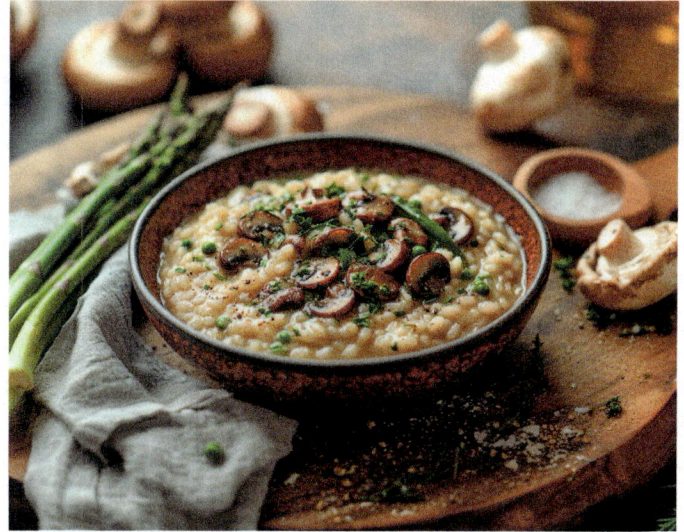

Mushroom and asparagus risotto

Prep: 10 minutes | Cook: 25 minutes | Serves:4

Ingredients:

- 1 cup brown rice (180g)
- 1 cup mushrooms, sliced (150g)
- 1 cup asparagus, chopped (150g)
- 4 cups vegetable broth (960ml)
- 1 tbsp olive oil (15ml)
- 1/4 tsp salt (1g)
- 1/4 tsp black pepper

Instructions:

1. Heat olive oil in a large pan over medium heat. Add mushrooms and sauté for 5 minutes until soft.
2. Add rice to the pan and stir for 2-3 minutes.
3. Gradually add vegetable broth, one cup at a time, allowing the rice to absorb the liquid before adding more. Stir frequently.
4. When the rice is nearly cooked, add the chopped asparagus, salt, and pepper. Cook for another 5 minutes until the rice is tender and the asparagus is bright green.
5. Serve warm.

Nutritional Facts (Per Serving): Calories: 476 | Protein: 14g | Fat: 11g | Carbs: 45g | Fiber: 7g | Sodium: 530mg | Sugars: 6g

CHAPTER 10: LUNCHES: Healthy dishes from cereals and legumes

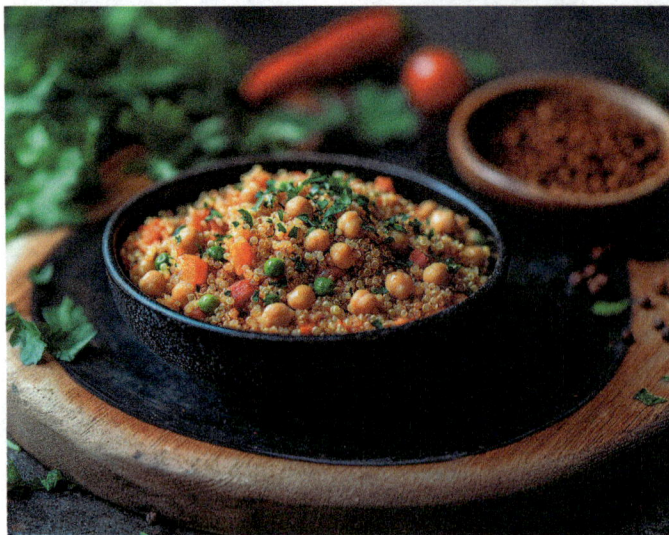

Chickpea and quinoa pilaf

Prep: 10 minutes | Cook: 20 minutes | Serves:4

Ingredients:

- 1 cup quinoa (170g)
- 1 cup cooked chickpeas (240g)
- 1/2 cup diced carrots (75g)
- 1/2 cup peas (75g)
- 4 cups vegetable broth (960ml)
- 1 tbsp olive oil (15ml)
- 1/4 tsp salt
- 1/4 tsp black pepper

Instructions:

1. Heat olive oil in a pot over medium heat. Add carrots and sauté for 5 minutes.
2. Add quinoa, chickpeas, peas, vegetable broth, salt, and pepper. Bring to a boil.
3. Reduce heat, cover, and simmer for 15 minutes until quinoa is tender.
4. Serve warm.

Nutritional Facts (Per Serving): Calories: 497 | Protein: 16g | Fat: 11g | Carbs: 45g | Fiber: 7g | Sodium: 520mg | Sugars: 6g

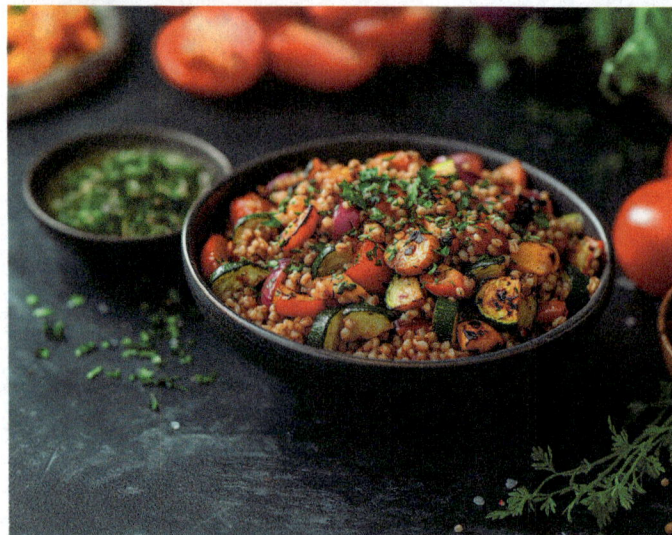

Farro and roasted vegetable bowl

Prep: 15 minutes | Cook: 25 minutes | Serves:4

Ingredients:

- 1 cup farro (200g)
- 1 cup zucchini, diced (150g)
- 1 cup bell peppers, diced (150g)
- 1 onion, sliced (120g)
- 1 tbsp olive oil (15ml)
- 4 cups vegetable broth (960ml)
- 1/4 tsp salt
- 1/4 tsp black pepper

Instructions:

1. Preheat oven to 400°F (200°C). Toss zucchini, bell peppers, and onions with olive oil, salt, and pepper. Roast for 20 minutes.
2. Cook farro in vegetable broth according to package instructions.
3. Mix the roasted vegetables with cooked farro and serve warm.

Nutritional Facts (Per Serving): Calories: 492 | Protein: 14g | Fat: 12g | Carbs: 46g | Fiber: 7g | Sodium: 530mg | Sugars: 6g

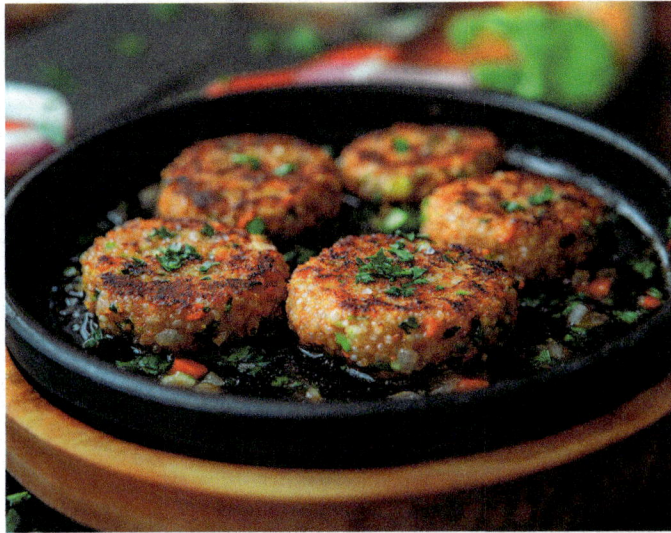

Amaranth veggie patties

Prep: 15 minutes | Cook: 20 minutes | Serves:4

Ingredients:

- 1 cup amaranth (190g)
- 1/2 cup grated carrots (75g)
- 1/2 cup grated zucchini (75g)
- 1/4 cup diced onions (40g)
- 1 tbsp olive oil (15ml)
- 4 cups vegetable broth (960ml)
- 1/4 tsp salt
- 1/4 tsp black pepper

Instructions:

1. Cook amaranth in vegetable broth according to package instructions.
2. Mix cooked amaranth with grated carrots, zucchini, onions, salt, and pepper. Form into patties.
3. Heat olive oil in a pan over medium heat and cook patties for 3-4 minutes per side until golden.
4. Serve warm.

Nutritional Facts (Per Serving): Calories: 476 | Protein: 15g | Fat: 11g | Carbs: 45g | Fiber: 8g | Sodium: 540mg | Sugars: 5g

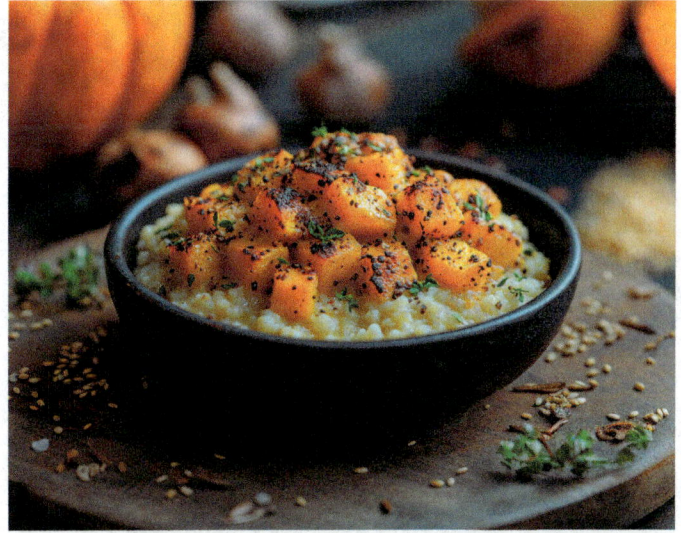

Bowl of millet and baked pumpkin with cheese sauce

Prep: 10 minutes | Cook: 30 minutes | Serves:4

Ingredients:

- 1 cup millet (200g)
- 2 cups diced pumpkin (300g)
- 1/2 cup shredded low-fat cheddar cheese (60g)
- 1/2 cup almond milk (120ml)
- 1 tbsp olive oil (15ml)
- 1/4 tsp salt
- 1/4 tsp black pepper
- 1/4 tsp garlic powder

Instructions:

1. Preheat the oven to 400°F (200°C). Toss diced pumpkin with olive oil, salt, and pepper, then roast for 25 minutes until tender.
2. Cook millet in 2 cups of water (480ml) for 15-20 minutes until tender and water is absorbed.
3. In a small saucepan, heat almond milk and stir in shredded cheese and garlic powder. Cook until the cheese is melted and the sauce is smooth.
4. Serve the cooked millet in bowls, top with roasted pumpkin, and drizzle with the cheese sauce.

Nutritional Facts (Per Serving): Calories: 469 | Protein: 16g | Fat: 11g | Carbs: 45g | Fiber: 7g | Sodium: 530mg | Sugars: 6g

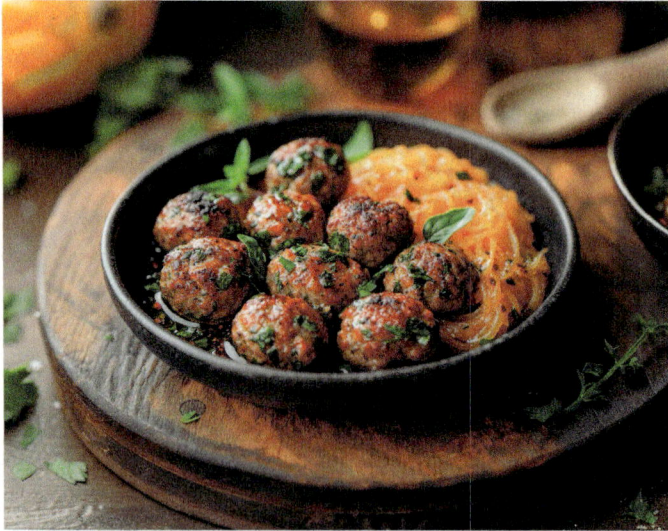

Turkey meatballs with spaghetti squash

Prep: 15 minutes | Cook: 30 minutes | Serves:4

Ingredients:

- 1 lb ground turkey (450g)
- 1 egg, beaten
- 1/2 cup breadcrumbs (60g)
- 1 tsp garlic powder
- 1 tsp Italian seasoning
- 1/4 tsp salt
- 1 medium spaghetti squash (900g)
- 1 tbsp olive oil (15ml)

Instructions:

1. Preheat oven to 400°F (200°C). Cut spaghetti squash in half, drizzle with olive oil, and bake for 25-30 minutes until tender.
2. In a bowl, mix ground turkey, egg, breadcrumbs, garlic powder, Italian seasoning, and salt. Form into meatballs.
3. Bake the meatballs for 20 minutes or until cooked through.
4. Use a fork to scrape the spaghetti squash into strands, and serve with the turkey meatballs.

Nutritional Facts (Per Serving): Calories: 486 | Protein: 18g | Fat: 11g | Carbs: 46g | Fiber: 7g | Sodium: 530mg | Sugars: 6g

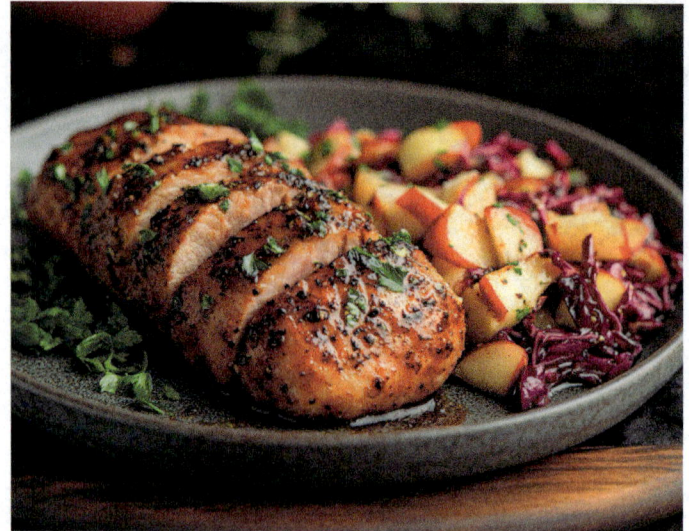

Pork tenderloin with apple slaw

Prep: 15 minutes | Cook: 25 minutes | Serves:4

Ingredients:

- 1 lb pork tenderloin (450g)
- 1 tbsp olive oil (15ml)
- 1/4 tsp salt
- 1/4 tsp black pepper
- 2 apples, julienned (240g)
- 2 cups shredded cabbage (150g)
- 1 tbsp apple cider vinegar (15ml)
- 1 tsp honey (7g)

Instructions:

1. Preheat oven to 375°F (190°C). Season pork tenderloin with olive oil, salt, and pepper. Bake for 25 minutes until cooked through.
2. In a bowl, mix apples, cabbage, apple cider vinegar, and honey to make the slaw.
3. Slice the pork and serve with the apple slaw.

Nutritional Facts (Per Serving): Calories: 497 | Protein: 19g | Fat: 12g | Carbs: 45g | Fiber: 6g | Sodium: 520mg | Sugars: 7g

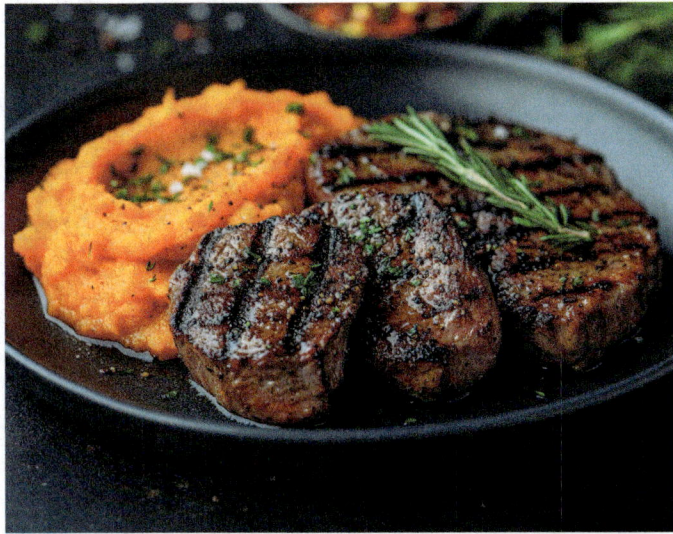

Lamb chops with sweet potato mash

Prep: 10 minutes | Cook: 30 minutes | Serves:4

Ingredients:

- 4 lamb chops (400g)
- 2 medium sweet potatoes (400g)
- 1 tbsp olive oil (15ml)
- 1/2 tsp rosemary, chopped
- 1/4 tsp salt
- 1/4 tsp black pepper

Instructions:

1. Preheat grill to medium heat. Season lamb chops with olive oil, rosemary, salt, and pepper. Grill for 4-5 minutes per side until cooked through.
2. Meanwhile, boil sweet potatoes until soft, mash them, and season with salt and pepper.
3. Serve the lamb chops with the sweet potato mash.

Nutritional Facts (Per Serving): Calories: 502 | Protein: 17g | Fat: 13g | Carbs: 44g | Fiber: 6g | Sodium: 530mg | Sugars: 6g

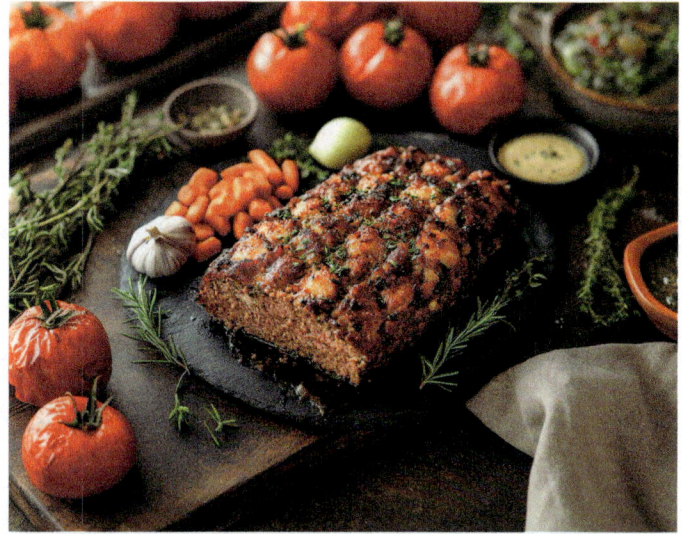

Lean beef and lamb meatloaf with herbs and vegetables

Prep: 15 minutes | Cook: 45 minutes | Serves:4

Ingredients:

- 1/2 lb lean ground beef (225g)
- 1/2 lb ground lamb (225g)
- 1/2 cup diced carrots (75g)
- 1/2 cup diced onions (75g)
- 1/2 cup breadcrumbs (60g)
- 1 egg, beaten
- 1 tsp mixed herbs (thyme, rosemary)
- 1/4 tsp salt
- 1/4 tsp black pepper

Instructions:

1. Preheat oven to 375°F (190°C). In a bowl, combine beef, lamb, carrots, onions, breadcrumbs, egg, herbs, salt, and pepper.
2. Form the mixture into a loaf and place it in a baking dish.
3. Bake for 45 minutes or until cooked through.
4. Let rest for 5 minutes before slicing.

Nutritional Facts (Per Serving): Calories: 497 | Protein: 19g | Fat: 13g | Carbs: 45g | Fiber: 7g | Sodium: 520mg | Sugars: 6g

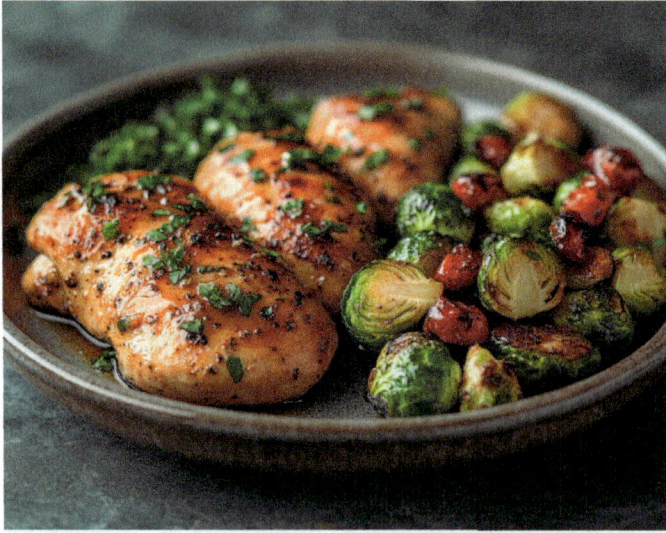

Honey mustard chicken with roasted Brussels sprouts

Prep: 10 minutes | Cook: 30 minutes | Serves:4

Ingredients:

- 1 lb chicken breasts, boneless (450g)
- 1 tbsp honey (21g)
- 1 tbsp Dijon mustard (15g)
- 1 tbsp olive oil (15ml)
- 2 cups Brussels sprouts, halved (300g)
- 1/4 tsp salt
- 1/4 tsp black pepper

Instructions:

1. Preheat oven to 400°F (200°C). Toss Brussels sprouts with olive oil, salt, and pepper, and roast for 20 minutes.
2. In a small bowl, mix honey and mustard. Brush the chicken breasts with the honey mustard mixture.
3. Roast the chicken alongside the Brussels sprouts for an additional 10 minutes until fully cooked.
4. Serve warm.

Nutritional Facts (Per Serving): Calories: 486 | Protein: 18g | Fat: 11g | Carbs: 46g | Fiber: 7g | Sodium: 510mg | Sugars: 7g

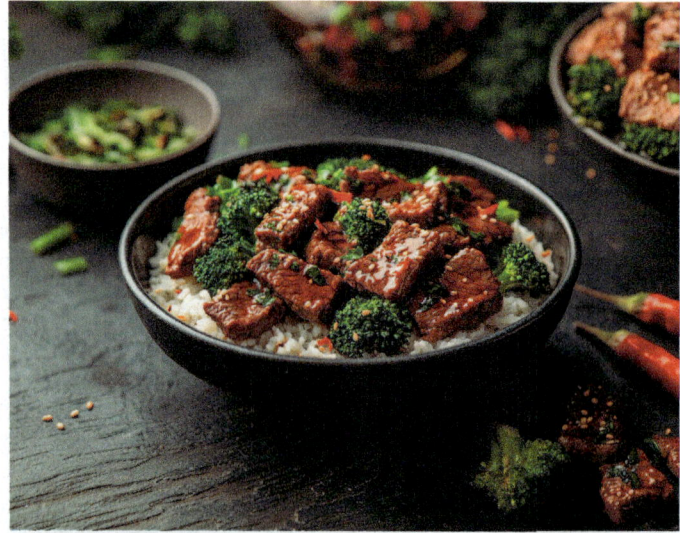

Asian-style boiled lenten beef and broccoli with wild rice

Prep: 10 minutes | Cook: 30 minutes | Serves:4

Ingredients:

- 1/2 lb lean beef, sliced (225g)
- 2 cups broccoli florets (300g)
- 1 cup wild rice (180g)
- 4 cups vegetable broth (960ml)
- 1 tbsp soy sauce (15ml)
- 1 tsp ginger, minced
- 1 tbsp olive oil (15ml)

Instructions:

1. In a pot, bring vegetable broth to a boil and cook wild rice according to package instructions.
2. In a separate pot, heat olive oil and sauté ginger for 2 minutes. Add beef slices and cook until browned.
3. Add broccoli and soy sauce to the beef, cover, and simmer for 10 minutes until broccoli is tender.
4. Serve the beef and broccoli over wild rice.

Nutritional Facts (Per Serving): Calories: 475 | Protein: 16g | Fat: 12g | Carbs: 45g | Fiber: 8g | Sodium: 530mg | Sugars: 6g

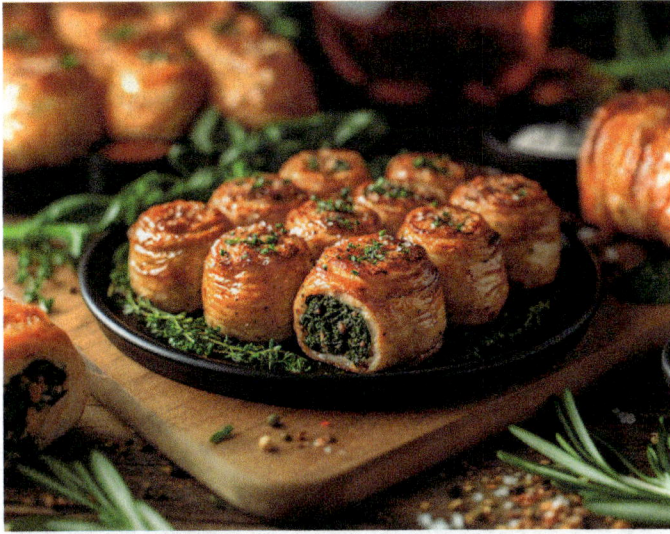

Turkey and spinach mini rolls

Prep: 15 minutes | Cook: 25 minutes | Serves:4

Ingredients:

- 1 lb ground turkey (450g)
- 1 cup fresh spinach, finely chopped (30g)
- 1/2 cup breadcrumbs (60g)
- 1 egg, beaten
- 1 tsp dried thyme
- 1/4 tsp salt
- 1/4 tsp black pepper

Instructions:

1. Preheat the oven to 375°F (190°C). In a bowl, mix ground turkey, spinach, breadcrumbs, egg, thyme, salt, and pepper.
2. Form the mixture into small rolls and place on a baking sheet.
3. Bake for 20-25 minutes until golden brown and fully cooked.
4. Serve warm.

Nutritional Facts (Per Serving): Calories: 490 | Protein: 18g | Fat: 11g | Carbs: 46g | Fiber: 7g | Sodium: 520mg | Sugars: 6g

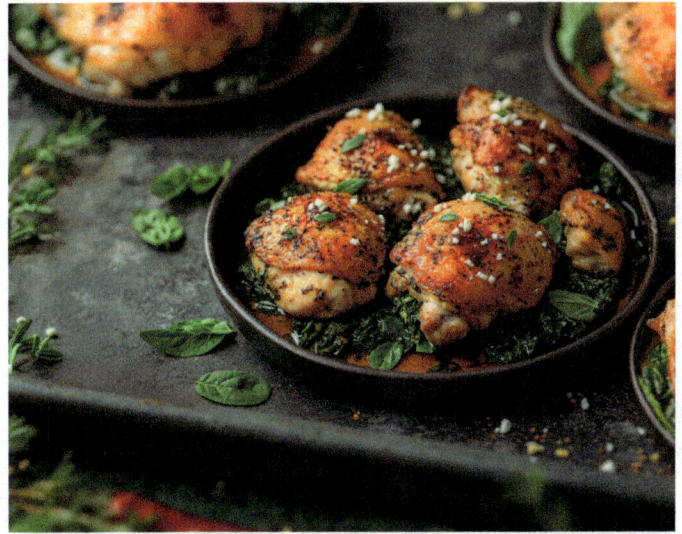

Spinach and feta stuffed chicken thighs

Prep: 15 minutes | Cook: 35 minutes | Serves:4

Ingredients:

- 4 chicken thighs, boneless (500g)
- 1/2 cup feta cheese, crumbled (100g)
- 1 cup fresh spinach, chopped (30g)
- 1 tbsp olive oil (15ml)
- 1/4 tsp salt
- 1/4 tsp black pepper

Instructions:

1. Preheat the oven to 375°F (190°C). In a bowl, mix spinach and feta cheese.
2. Stuff each chicken thigh with the spinach-feta mixture and secure with toothpicks.
3. Place the chicken in a baking dish, drizzle with olive oil, and season with salt and pepper.
4. Bake for 30-35 minutes until the chicken is fully cooked.
5. Serve warm.

Nutritional Facts (Per Serving): Calories: 479 | Protein: 19g | Fat: 13g | Carbs: 42g | Fiber: 6g | Sodium: 530mg | Sugars: 5g

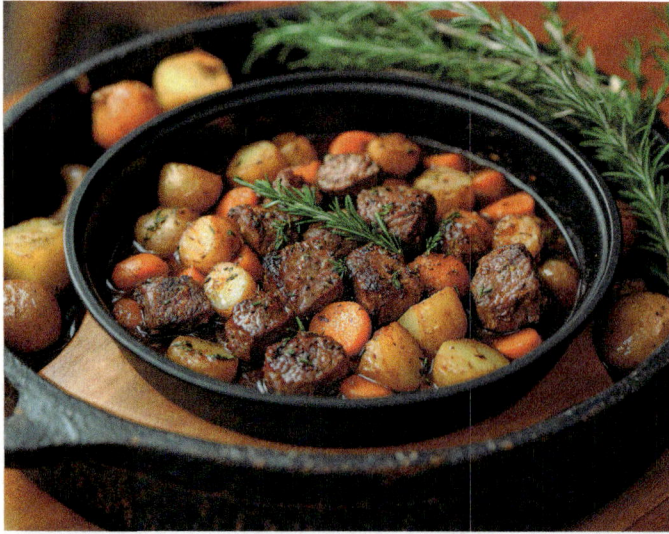

Braised lamb with rosemary and vegetables

Prep: 15 minutes | Cook: 1 hour 30 minutes | Serves: 4

Ingredients:

- 1 lb lean lamb, cubed (450g)
- 2 carrots, diced (120g)
- 2 potatoes, diced (300g)
- 1 tbsp fresh rosemary, chopped (2g)
- 4 cups low-acid vegetable broth (960ml)
- 1 tbsp olive oil (15ml)
- 1/4 tsp salt
- 1/4 tsp black pepper

Instructions:

1. Heat olive oil in a large pot over medium heat. Brown the lamb pieces for 5 minutes.

2. Add carrots, potatoes, rosemary, salt, and pepper to the pot. Stir for 2 minutes.

3. Pour in the broth, cover, and simmer on low heat for 1 hour 30 minutes until the lamb is tender.

4. Serve warm.

Nutritional Facts (Per Serving): Calories: 487 | Protein: 18g | Fat: 12g | Carbs: 45g | Fiber: 7g | Sodium: 530mg | Sugars: 6g

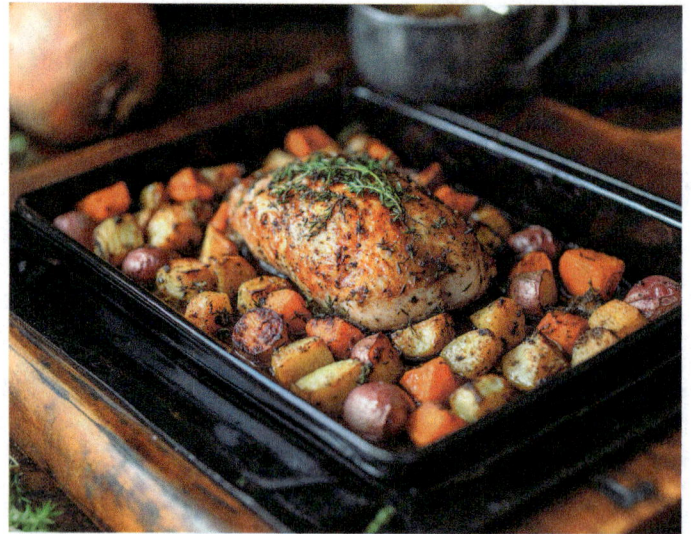

Herb-roasted turkey with vegetables

Prep: 15 minutes | Cook: 40 minutes | Serves:4

Ingredients:

- 1 lb turkey breast, cut into pieces (450g)
- 2 carrots, diced (120g)
- 1 parsnip, diced (150g)
- 1 sweet potato, diced (200g)
- 1 tbsp olive oil (15ml)
- 1 tbsp mixed herbs (rosemary, thyme, oregano) (2g)
- 1/4 tsp salt
- 1/4 tsp black pepper

Instructions:

1. Preheat oven to 375°F (190°C). Toss turkey, carrots, parsnip, and sweet potato with olive oil, herbs, salt, and pepper.

2. Spread the mixture on a baking sheet and roast for 35-40 minutes until the turkey is cooked through and the vegetables are tender.

3. Serve warm.

Nutritional Facts (Per Serving): Calories: 495 | Protein: 19g | Fat: 11g | Carbs: 45g | Fiber: 7g | Sodium: 510mg | Sugars: 5g

CHAPTER 12: SNACKS: Light bites and Low-Acid finger foods for any time

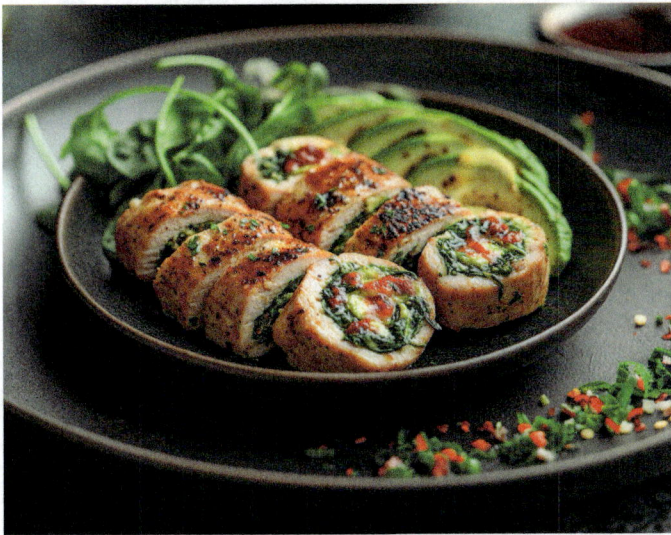

Avocado and turkey roll-ups

Prep: 10 minutes | Cook: 5 minutes | Serves: 2

Ingredients:

- 4 slices turkey breast (100g)
- 1/2 avocado, mashed (75g)
- 1/2 cup fresh spinach (15g)
- 1 tsp lemon juice (5ml)

Instructions:

1. Lay out the turkey slices: Place each turkey slice flat on a clean surface. Spread a small amount of Dijon mustard (about 1/4 tsp) on each slice to add flavor.
2. Add the avocado and spinach: Place 1-2 slices of avocado and a few spinach leaves on one end of each turkey slice. Ensure the filling is distributed evenly.
3. Roll up the turkey slices: Starting from the end with the avocado and spinach, carefully roll each turkey slice into a tight roll. Ensure the filling is securely tucked inside.
4. Serve: Slice each roll-up in half if desired or serve whole for a light and refreshing meal.

Nutritional Facts (Per Serving): Calories: 210 | Protein: 9g | Fat: 6g | Carbs: 8g | Fiber: 3g | Sodium: 320mg | Sugars: 4g

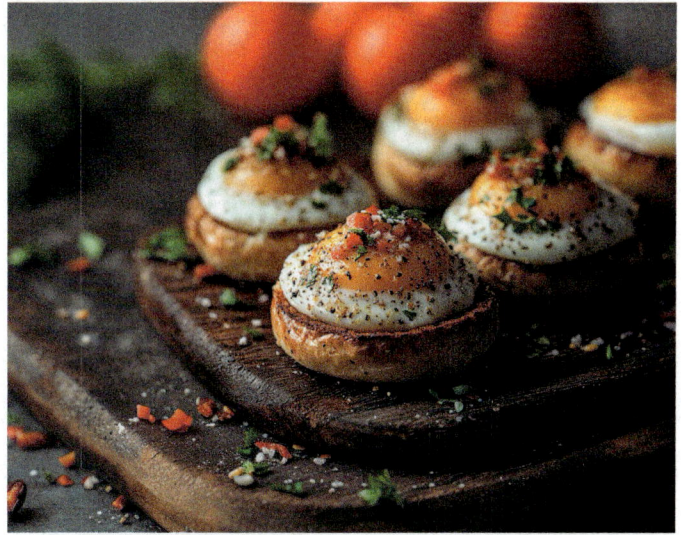

Eggs baked in small buns with bell peppers

Prep: 10 minutes | Cook: 15 minutes | Serves:2

Ingredients:

- 2 small whole-wheat buns (120g)
- 2 eggs
- 1/4 cup diced bell peppers (40g)
- 1 tbsp shredded low-fat cheddar cheese (15g)
- 1/4 tsp salt

Instructions:

1. Preheat the oven to 375°F (190°C). Hollow out the center of each bun.
2. Crack an egg into each bun, top with diced bell peppers and cheese, and season with salt.
3. Bake for 12-15 minutes until the eggs are set.
4. Serve warm.

Nutritional Facts (Per Serving): Calories: 216 | Protein: 10g | Fat: 6g | Carbs: 20g | Fiber: 2g | Sodium: 330mg | Sugars: 5g

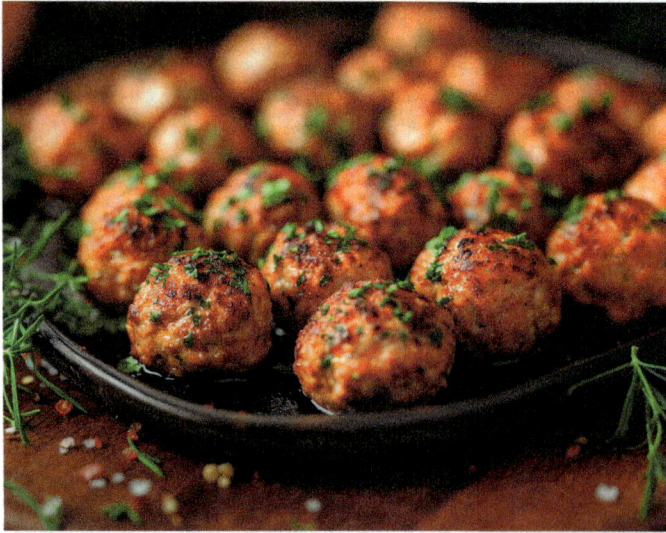

Mini chicken meatballs

Prep: 10 minutes | Cook: 20 minutes | Serves:2

Ingredients:

- 1/2 lb ground chicken (225g)
- 1/4 cup breadcrumbs (30g)
- 1 tbsp fresh parsley, chopped (2g)
- 1 egg, beaten
- 1 tsp garlic powder
- 1/4 tsp salt

Instructions:

1. Preheat the oven to 400°F (200°C). In a bowl, mix chicken, breadcrumbs, parsley, egg, garlic powder, and salt.
2. Form into small meatballs and place on a baking sheet.
3. Bake for 18-20 minutes until golden brown and fully cooked.
4. Serve warm.

Nutritional Facts (Per Serving): Calories: 221 | Protein: 10g | Fat: 6g | Carbs: 20g | Fiber: 1g | Sodium: 340mg | Sugars: 5g

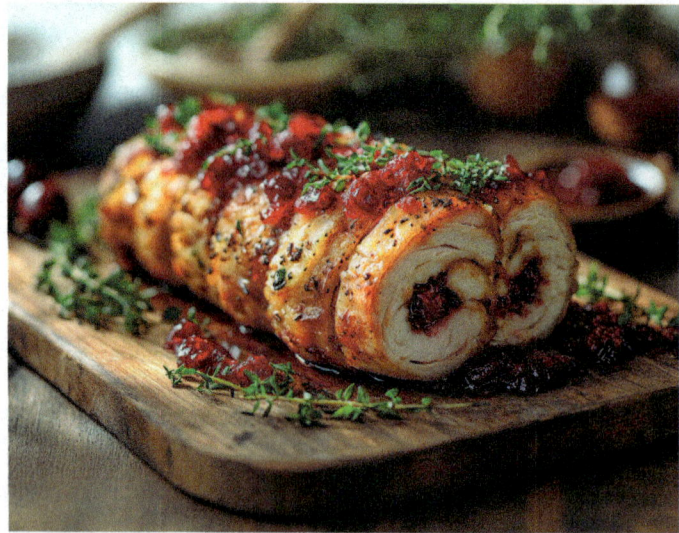

Turkey and cranberry pinwheels

Prep: 10 minutes | Cook: 5 minutes | Serves: 2

Ingredients:

- 2 whole wheat tortillas (120g)
- 4 tbsp cranberry sauce (60g)
- 4 slices turkey breast (100g)
- 1/2 cup fresh spinach (15g)

Instructions:

1. Prepare the tortillas: Lay the tortillas flat on a clean surface and evenly spread 1 tbsp of cranberry sauce on each.
2. Layer the turkey and spinach: Place 2 slices of turkey breast and a handful of spinach leaves on each tortilla, spreading them evenly.
3. Roll and slice: Roll up each tortilla tightly, then slice into 1-inch pinwheels.
4. Serve: Arrange the pinwheels on a plate and serve fresh.

Nutritional Facts (Per Serving): Calories: 215 | Protein: 10g | Fat: 6g | Carbs: 22g | Fiber: 2g | Sodium: 320mg | Sugars: 6g

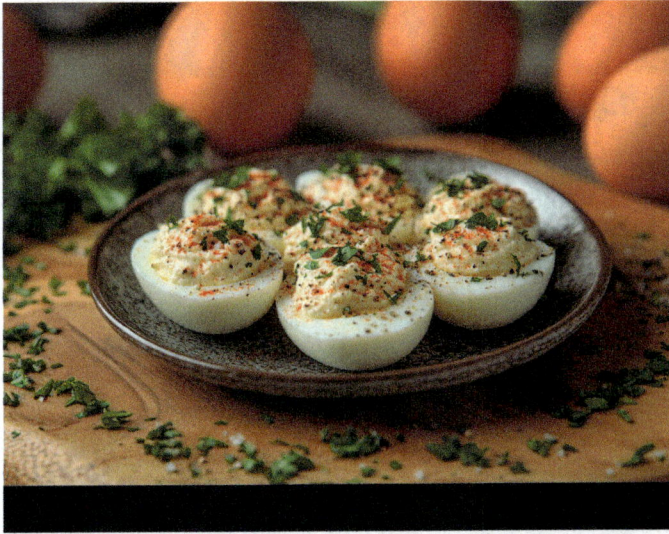

Ricotta and herb-stuffed eggs

Prep: 10 minutes | Cook: 10 minutes | Serves:2

Ingredients:

- 4 hard-boiled eggs, halved (200g)
- 1/4 cup ricotta cheese (60g)
- 1 tbsp fresh parsley, chopped (2g)
- 1/4 tsp salt
- 1/4 tsp black pepper

Instructions:

1. Scoop out the yolks from the hard-boiled eggs and mix them with ricotta, parsley, salt, and pepper.
2. Spoon the ricotta mixture back into the egg whites.
3. Serve as a savory appetizer or snack.

Nutritional Facts (Per Serving): Calories: 200 | Protein: 9g | Fat: 6g | Carbs: 18g | Fiber: 1g | Sodium: 340mg | Sugars: 4g

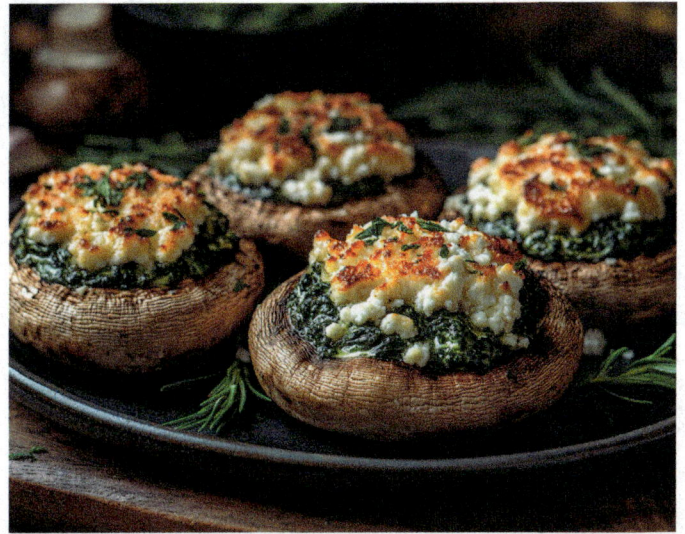

Spinach and feta stuffed mushrooms

Prep: 10 minutes | Cook: 15 minutes | Serves:2

Ingredients:

- 8 button mushrooms, stems removed (150g)
- 1/2 cup fresh spinach, chopped (15g)
- 1/4 cup crumbled feta cheese (50g)
- 1 tbsp olive oil (15ml)

Instructions:

1. Preheat the oven to 375°F (190°C). In a bowl, mix spinach and feta cheese.
2.Stuff each mushroom cap with the spinach-feta mixture.
3.Drizzle with olive oil and bake for 12-15 minutes until golden and tender.
4. Serve warm as an appetizer.

Nutritional Facts (Per Serving):Calories: 211 | Protein: 7g | Fat: 7g | Carbs: 21g | Fiber: 2g | Sodium: 330mg | Sugars: 5g

CHAPTER 13: SNACKS: Homemade pates, sauces and spreads

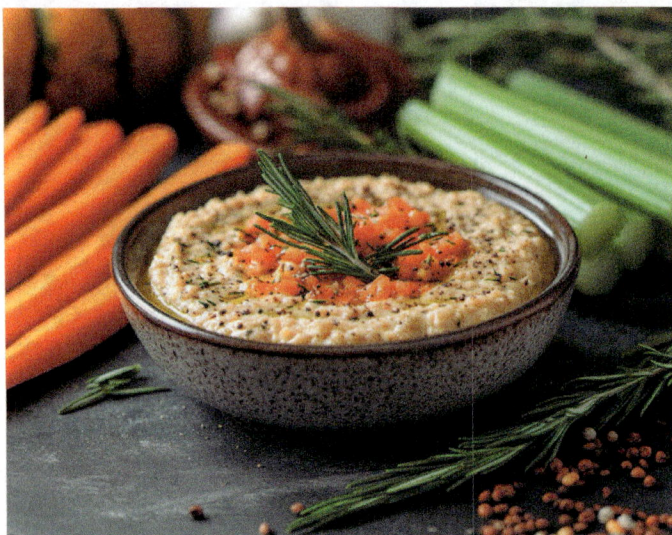

White bean and rosemary pate

Prep: 10 minutes | Cook: 20 minutes | Serves:2

Ingredients:

- 1 cup cooked white beans (240g)
- 1 tbsp fresh rosemary, chopped (2g)
- 1 tbsp olive oil (15ml)
- 1/2 tsp garlic powder
- 1/4 tsp salt
- 1/2 cup carrot sticks (60g)
- 1/2 cup celery sticks (60g)
- 1/2 cup pumpkin sticks (60g)

Instructions:

1. Sauté garlic and rosemary: Heat olive oil in a pan and sauté garlic and rosemary for 2-3 minutes.
2. Blend: Combine the sautéed mixture with white beans, lemon juice, salt, and pepper in a blender. Blend until smooth.
3. Serve: Adjust consistency with water if needed and serve with vegetables or crackers.

Nutritional Facts (Per Serving): Calories: 217 | Protein: 9g | Fat: 6g | Carbs: 22g | Fiber: 3g | Sodium: 340mg | Sugars: 5g

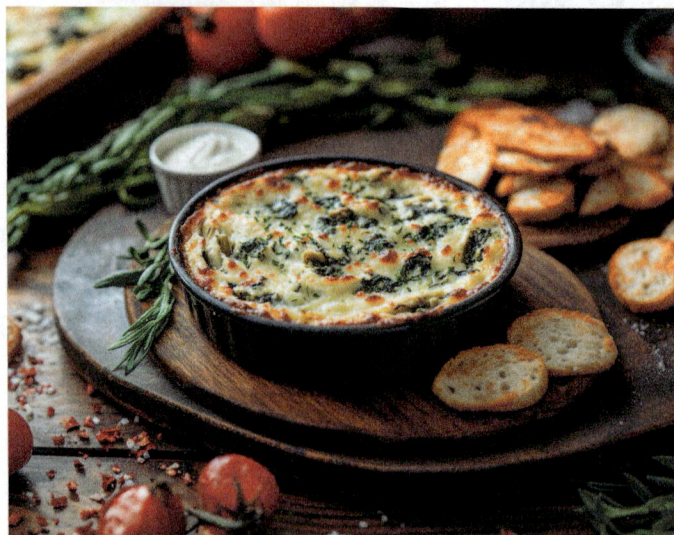

Spinach and artichoke dip

Prep: 10 minutes | Cook: 15 minutes | Serves:2

Ingredients:

- 1/2 cup fresh spinach, chopped (15g)
- 1/2 cup canned artichoke hearts, chopped (75g)
- 1/2 cup Greek yogurt (120g)
- 1/4 cup shredded low-fat mozzarella (30g)
- 1/4 tsp garlic powder
- 1/4 tsp salt

Instructions:

1. Preheat oven to 375°F (190°C). Mix spinach, artichokes, Greek yogurt, mozzarella, garlic powder, and salt.
2. Transfer to a baking dish and bake for 12-15 minutes until bubbly.
3. Serve warm.

Nutritional Facts (Per Serving): Calories: 213 | Protein: 9g | Fat: 7g | Carbs: 20g | Fiber: 2g | Sodium: 330mg | Sugars: 4g

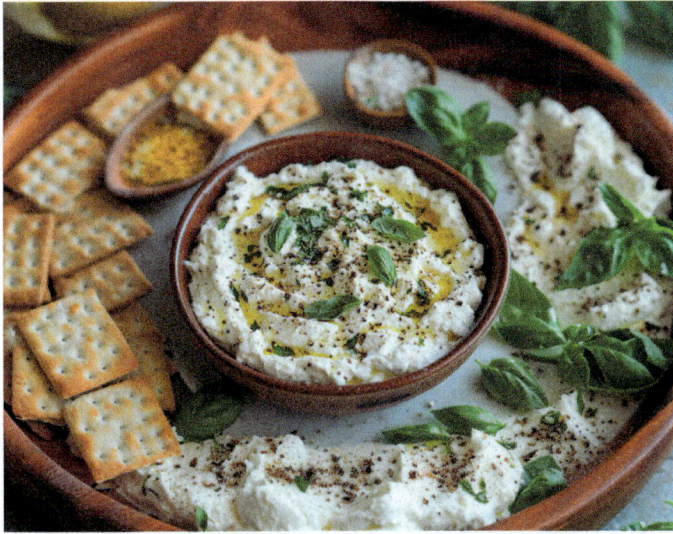

Basil and ricotta spread

Prep: 5 minutes | Cook: 5 minutes | Serves: 2

Ingredients:

- 1/2 cup ricotta cheese (120g)
- 1 tbsp fresh basil, chopped (2g)
- 1 tsp lemon juice (5ml)
- 1/4 tsp salt
- 1/4 tsp black pepper

Instructions:

1. Mix ricotta, basil, lemon juice, salt, and pepper until smooth.
2. Serve with crackers or vegetable sticks.

Nutritional Facts (Per Serving): Calories: 219 | Protein: 10g | Fat: 6g | Carbs: 20g | Fiber: 1g | Sodium: 320mg | Sugars: 5g

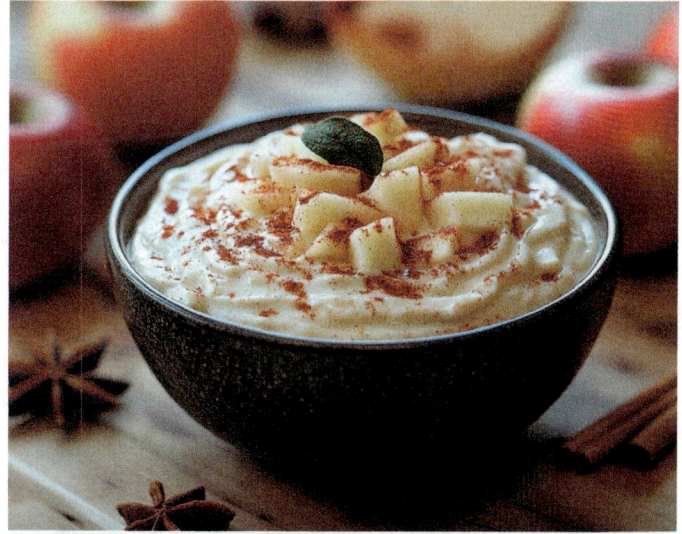

Apple and cinnamon yogurt dip

Prep: 5 minutes | Cook: 5 minutes | Serves: 2

Ingredients:

- 1 cup Greek yogurt (240g)
- 1 small apple, finely diced (100g)
- 1/2 tsp ground cinnamon (2g)

Instructions:

1. Mix Greek yogurt, diced apple, and cinnamon in a bowl.
2. Serve chilled with lean turkey or chicken slices.

Nutritional Facts (Per Serving): Calories: 226 | Protein: 9g | Fat: 6g | Carbs: 22g | Fiber: 2g | Sodium: 320mg | Sugars: 6g

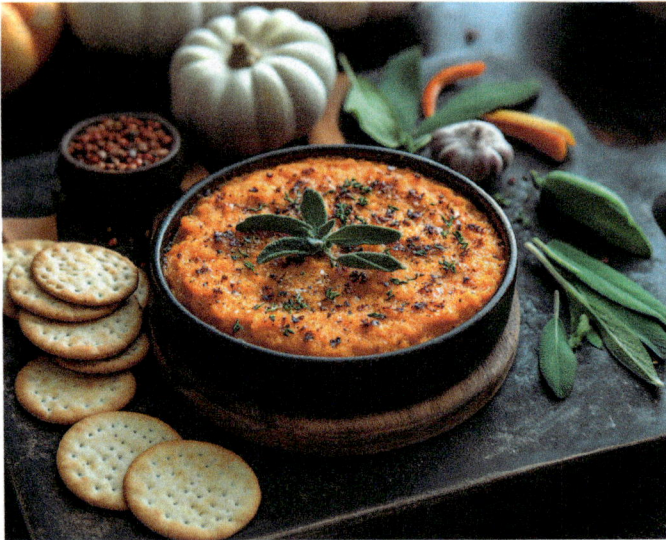

Pumpkin and sage spread

Prep: 10 minutes | Cook: 10 minutes | Serves:2

Ingredients:

- 1 cup pumpkin puree (240g)
- 1 tbsp fresh sage, chopped (2g)
- 1 clove garlic, minced
- 1 tbsp olive oil (15ml)

Instructions:

1. Heat olive oil in a pan over medium heat. Add garlic and sage, cook for 2 minutes.
2. Stir in pumpkin puree and cook for 5-7 minutes until warmed through.
3. Serve as a spread on crackers or vegetable sticks.

Nutritional Facts (Per Serving): Calories: 221 | Protein: 7g | Fat: 6g | Carbs: 24g | Fiber: 3g | Sodium: 330mg | Sugars: 5g

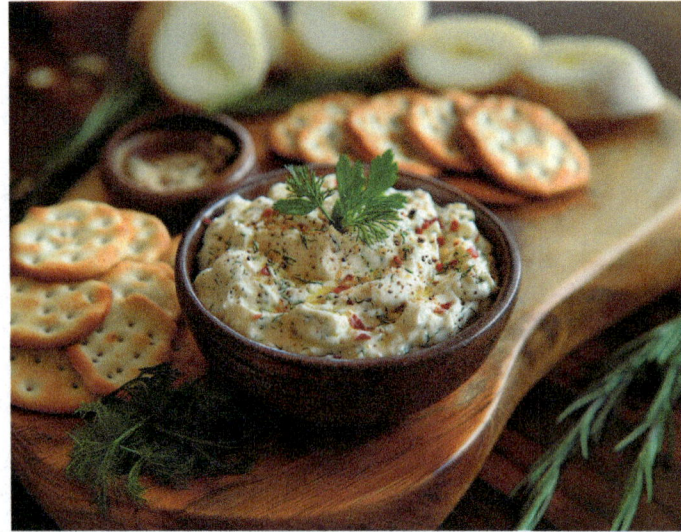

Herb cream cheese

Prep: 10 minutes | Cook: 5 minutes | Serves: 2

Ingredients:

- 1/2 cup low-fat cream cheese (120g)
- 1 tbsp fresh parsley, chopped (2g)
- 1 tsp fresh dill, chopped (1g)
- 1/4 tsp salt

Instructions:

1. Mix cream cheese, parsley, dill, and salt until well combined.
2. Serve as a spread on whole wheat crackers or as a dip for vegetables.

Nutritional Facts (Per Serving): Calories: 211 | Protein: 8g | Fat: 7g | Carbs: 18g | Fiber: 1g | Sodium: 340mg | Sugars: 4g

CHAPTER 14: DESSERTS: The right fruits, puddings and other goodies

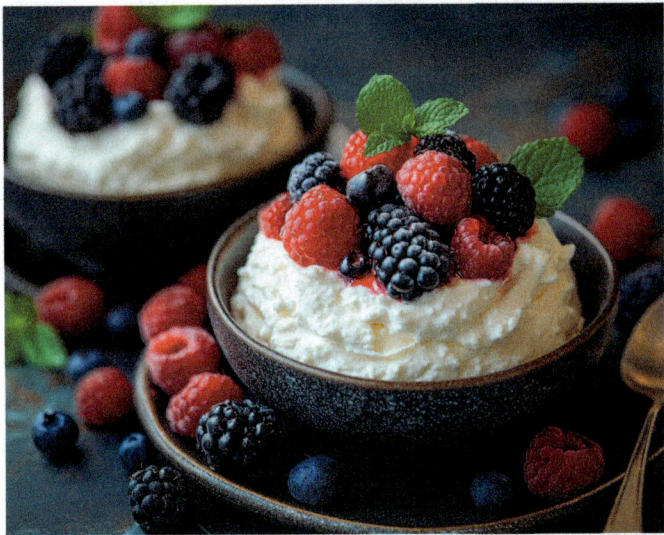

Cakes with whipped cottage cheese mousse and seasonal berries

Prep: 15 minutes | Cook: 10 minutes | Serves:2

Ingredients:

- 1/2 cup low-fat cottage cheese (120g)
- 1 tbsp honey (21g)
- 1/2 tsp vanilla extract (2g)
- 1/2 cup seasonal berries (75g)
- 2 whole wheat biscuits (60g)

Instructions:

1. Blend cottage cheese, honey, and vanilla extract until smooth and fluffy.
2. Spread the mousse over whole wheat biscuits and top with seasonal berries.
3. Serve immediately.

Nutritional Facts (Per Serving): Calories: 213 | Protein: 9g | Fat: 6g | Carbs: 25g | Fiber: 2g | Sodium: 320mg | Sugars: 6g

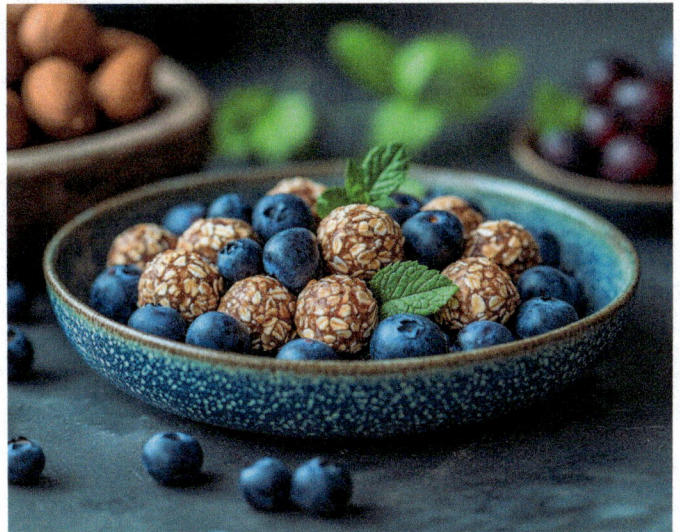

Blueberry and almond energy bites

Prep: 10 minutes | Cook: 5 minutes | Serves: 2

Ingredients:

- 1/4 cup oats (40g)
- 1/4 cup dried blueberries (30g)
- 2 tbsp almonds, chopped (20g)
- 1 tbsp almond butter (15g)
- 1 tbsp honey (21g)

Instructions:

1. Mix oats, dried blueberries, almonds, almond butter, and honey in a bowl.
2. Form into small bites and chill in the refrigerator for 20 minutes before serving.

Nutritional Facts (Per Serving): Calories: 215 | Protein: 8g | Fat: 7g | Carbs: 24g | Fiber: 3g | Sodium: 300mg | Sugars: 7g

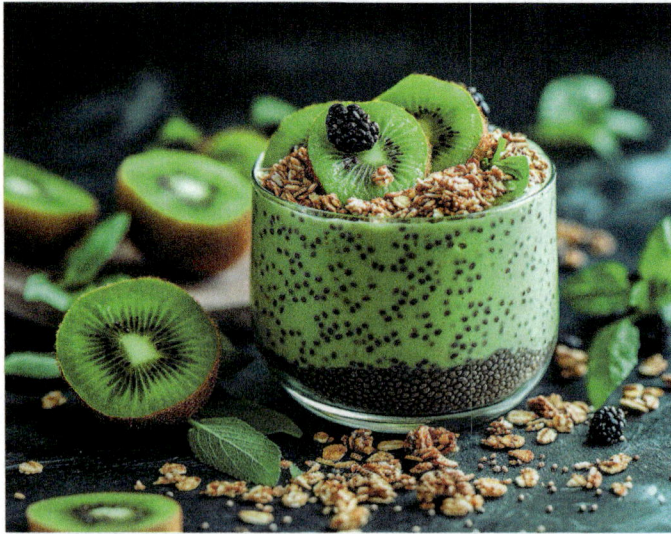

Kiwi and chia seed parfait

Prep: 10 minutes | Cook: 5 minutes | Serves: 2

Ingredients:

- 1 cup almond milk (240ml)
- 2 tbsp chia seeds (30g)
- 1 kiwi, sliced (80g)
- 2 tbsp granola (20g)

Instructions:

1. Mix chia seeds with almond milk and refrigerate for 30 minutes to thicken.
2. Layer chia pudding with kiwi slices and sprinkle with granola.
3. Serve immediately.

Nutritional Facts (Per Serving): Calories: 217 | Protein: 7g | Fat: 6g | Carbs: 24g | Fiber: 3g | Sodium: 310mg | Sugars: 5g

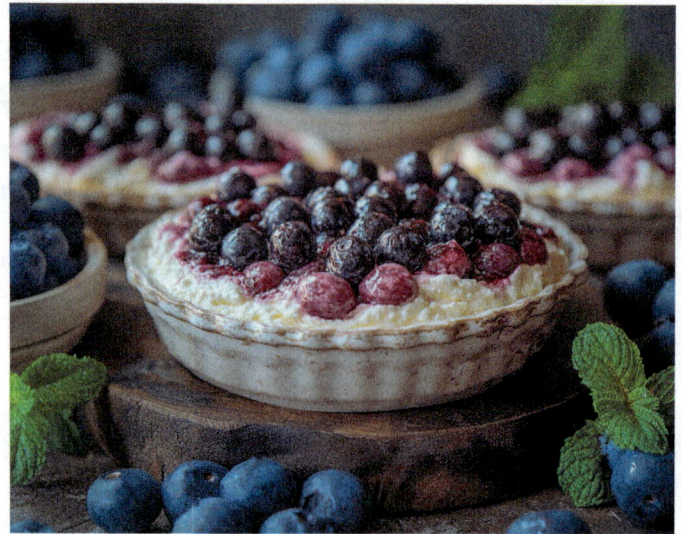

Curd casserole with blueberries and unsweetened cream

Prep: 10 minutes | Cook: 30 minutes | Serves:2

Ingredients:

- 1 cup low-fat cottage cheese (240g)
- 1/4 cup blueberries (40g)
- 1 tbsp honey (21g)
- 1 egg (50g)
- 1/2 tsp vanilla extract (2g)
- 2 tbsp unsweetened cream (30ml)

Instructions:

1. Preheat the oven to 350°F (180°C). Mix cottage cheese, honey, egg, and vanilla extract until smooth.
2. Fold in the blueberries and pour the mixture into a baking dish.
3. Bake for 25-30 minutes until set. Serve with a drizzle of unsweetened cream.

Nutritional Facts (Per Serving): Calories: 210 | Protein: 9g | Fat: 6g | Carbs: 22g | Fiber: 2g | Sodium: 320mg | Sugars: 5g

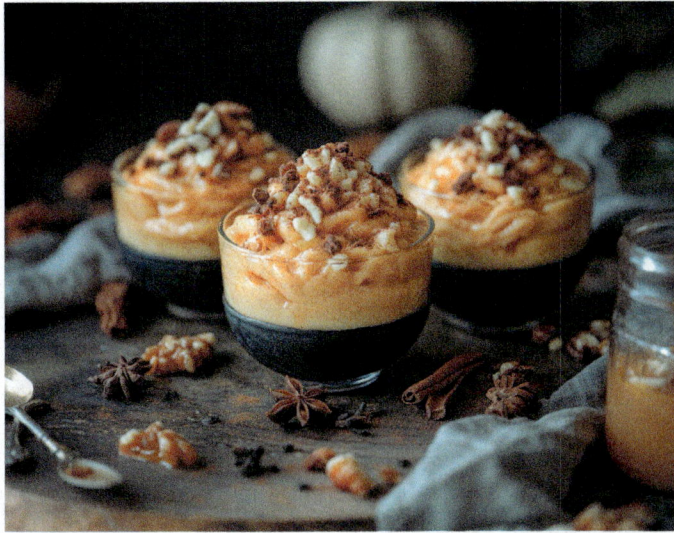

Pumpkin and coconut pudding

Prep: 10 minutes | Cook: 5 minutes | Serves: 2

Ingredients:

- 1 cup pumpkin puree (240g)
- 1/2 cup coconut milk (120ml)
- 1 tbsp honey (21g)
- 1/2 tsp ground cinnamon (2g)
- 1/4 tsp ground nutmeg

Instructions:

1. In a bowl, mix pumpkin puree, coconut milk, honey, cinnamon, and nutmeg.
2. Pour the mixture into small cups and chill for at least 1 hour until set.
3. Serve chilled.

Nutritional Facts (Per Serving): Calories: 215 | Protein: 7g | Fat: 7g | Carbs: 24g | Fiber: 2g | Sodium: 310mg | Sugars: 6g

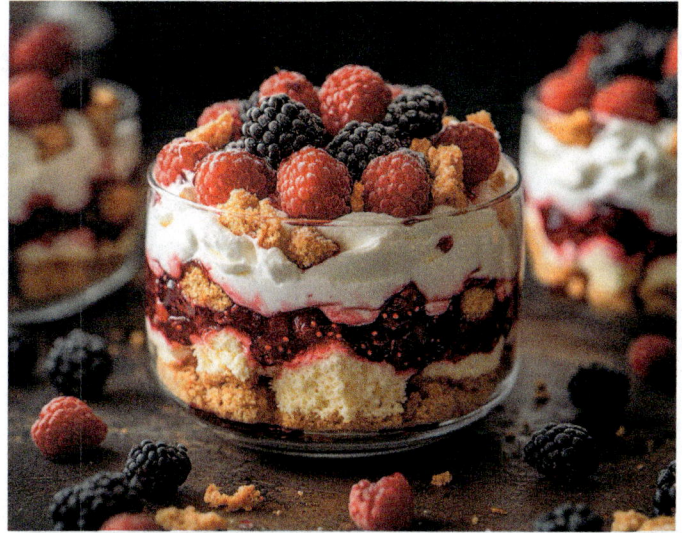

Trifle

Prep: 15 minutes | Cook: 10 minutes | Serves:2

Ingredients:

- 1 cup Greek yogurt (240g)
- 1/2 cup mixed berries (75g)
- 2 slices whole wheat sponge cake (60g)
- 1 tbsp honey (21g)

Instructions:

1. In serving glasses, layer pieces of sponge cake, Greek yogurt, and berries.
2. Drizzle with honey and repeat the layers.
3. Serve immediately or chill for a light, refreshing dessert.

Nutritional Facts (Per Serving): Calories: 200 | Protein: 9g | Fat: 5g | Carbs: 25g | Fiber: 3g | Sodium: 330mg | Sugars: 6g

CHAPTER 15: DESSERTS: Low-Acid cakes and bakes

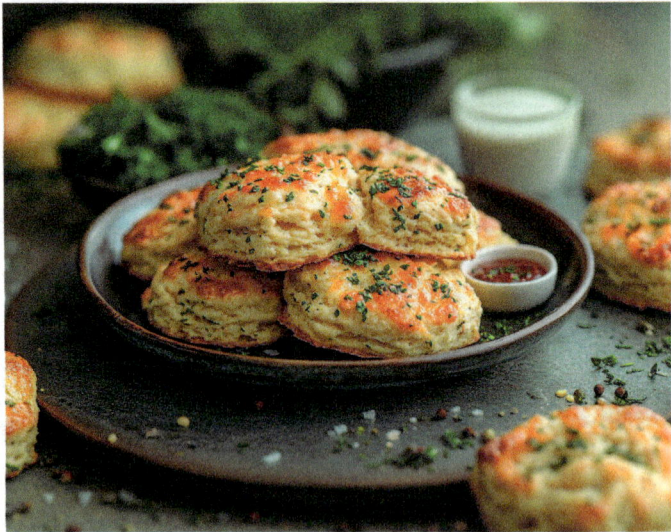

Herb and cheese scones

Prep: 10 minutes | Cook: 20 minutes | Serves:2

Ingredients:

- 1 cup whole wheat flour (120g)
- 1/4 cup shredded low-fat cheddar cheese (30g)
- 1 tbsp fresh herbs (e.g., parsley, thyme) (2g)
- 1 tsp baking powder (5g)
- 1/4 cup low-fat milk (60ml)
- 1 tbsp olive oil (15ml)

Instructions:

1. Preheat oven to 375°F (190°C). Mix flour, cheese, herbs, and baking powder in a bowl.
2. Add milk and olive oil, stirring until a dough forms.
3. Shape into small scones and bake for 15-20 minutes until golden.
4. Serve warm.

Nutritional Facts (Per Serving): Calories: 210 | Protein: 8g | Fat: 6g | Carbs: 22g | Fiber: 2g | Sodium: 340mg | Sugars: 4g

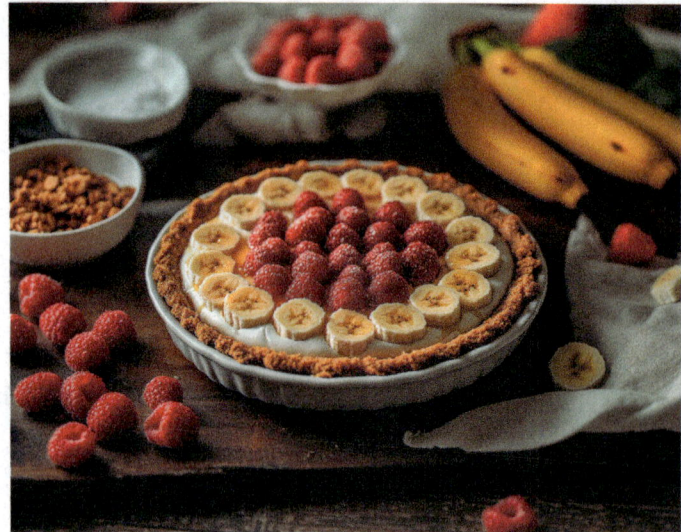

Banoffee pie

Prep: 15 minutes | Cook: 30 minutes | Serves:2

Ingredients:

- 1/2 cup mashed bananas (120g)
- 1/4 cup low-fat Greek yogurt (60g)
- 2 tbsp honey (21g)
- 1/4 cup whole wheat graham crackers, crushed (30g)
- 1 tbsp coconut oil (15ml)

Instructions:

1. Mix crushed graham crackers and melted coconut oil, pressing into a small dish to form a crust.
2. Layer with mashed bananas and Greek yogurt, then drizzle with honey.
3. Chill for 30 minutes before serving.

Nutritional Facts (Per Serving): Calories: 198 | Protein: 7g | Fat: 6g | Carbs: 26g | Fiber: 2g | Sodium: 320mg | Sugars: 6g

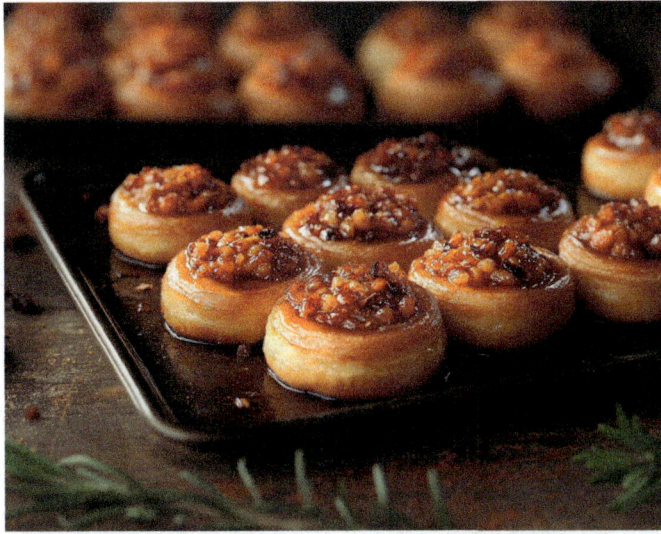

Low-acid chelsea buns

Prep: 15 minutes | Cook: 20 minutes | Serves:2

Ingredients:

- 1 cup whole wheat flour (120g)
- 1 tbsp honey (21g)
- 1/4 cup dried fruit (e.g., raisins, chopped apricots) (40g)
- 1 tsp cinnamon (5g)
- 1/2 cup almond milk (120ml)
- 1 tbsp olive oil (15ml)

Instructions:

1. Preheat oven to 350°F (180°C). Mix flour, cinnamon, and dried fruit.
2. Add almond milk, olive oil, and honey, stirring until a dough forms.
3. Roll dough into small buns and place on a baking sheet. Bake for 15-20 minutes until golden.
4. Serve warm.

Nutritional Facts (Per Serving): Calories: 216 | Protein: 8g | Fat: 5g | Carbs: 26g | Fiber: 3g | Sodium: 330mg | Sugars: 6g

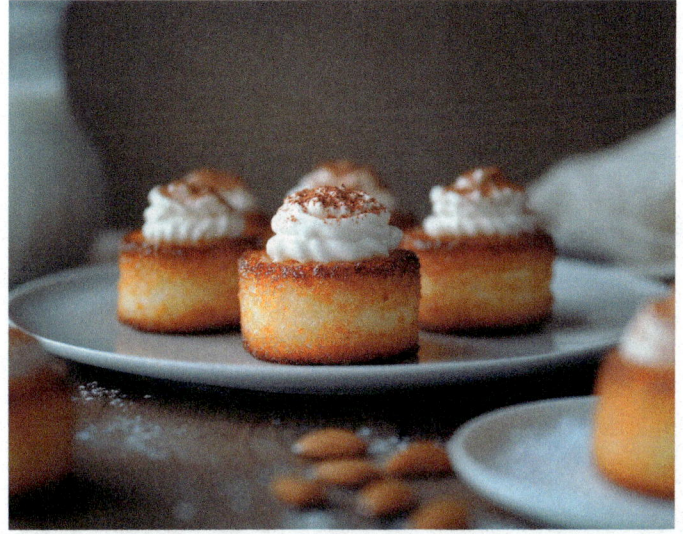

Low-acid twinkies

Prep: 15 minutes | Cook: 20 minutes | Serves:2

Ingredients:

- 1/2 cup whole wheat flour (60g)
- 1/4 tsp baking powder (1g)
- 1 tbsp honey (21g)
- 1/4 cup almond milk (60ml)
- 1/2 tsp vanilla extract (2g)
- 1/4 cup Greek yogurt (60g)

Instructions:

1. Preheat oven to 350°F (180°C). Mix flour, baking powder, honey, almond milk, and vanilla extract until smooth.
2. Pour into small molds and bake for 15-20 minutes.
3. Once cooled, fill with Greek yogurt.

Nutritional Facts (Per Serving): Calories: 191 | Protein: 8g | Fat: 6g | Carbs: 25g | Fiber: 2g | Sodium: 320mg | Sugars: 6g

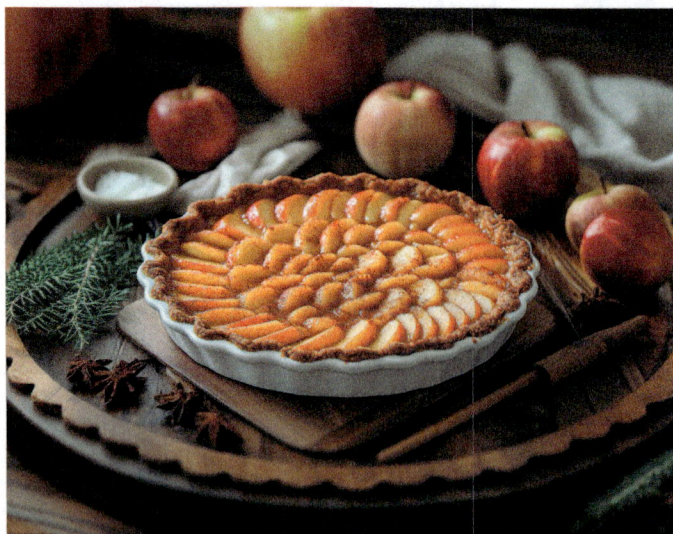

Low-acid american apple pie

Prep: 20 minutes | Cook: 30 minutes | Serves:2

Ingredients:

- 1 cup whole wheat flour (120g)
- 2 tbsp olive oil (30ml)
- 1 tbsp honey (21g)
- 1/2 tsp cinnamon (2g)
- 1 medium apple, sliced (150g)

Instructions:

1.Preheat oven to 375°F (190°C). Mix flour, olive oil, and a little water to form a dough. Roll out and place in a pie dish.
2. Layer apple slices over the crust, sprinkle with cinnamon and honey.
3. Bake for 25-30 minutes.

Nutritional Facts (Per Serving): Calories: 219 | Protein: 7g | Fat: 6g | Carbs: 26g | Fiber: 3g | Sodium: 300mg | Sugars: 6g

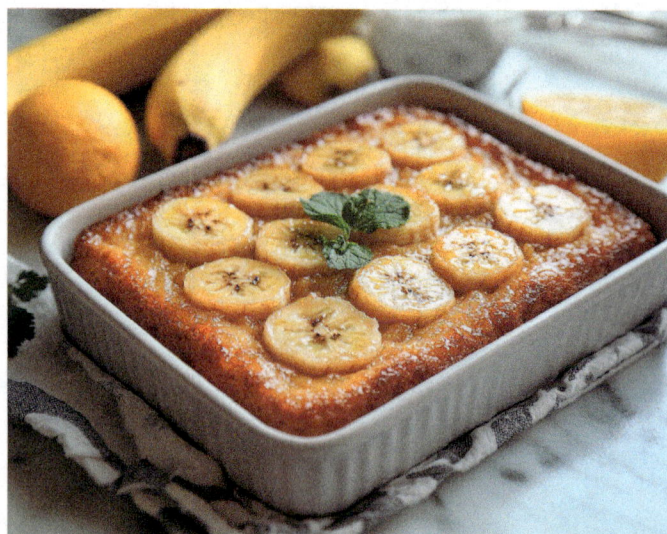

Low-acid banana cake

Prep: 15 minutes | Cook: 25 minutes | Serves:2

Ingredients:

- 1/2 cup mashed banana (120g)
- 1/2 cup whole wheat flour (60g)
- 1 tbsp honey (21g)
- 1/4 tsp baking soda (1g)
- 1/4 cup almond milk (60ml)

Instructions:

1. Preheat oven to 350°F (180°C). Mix mashed banana, flour, honey, baking soda, and almond milk.
2. Pour into a baking dish and bake for 20-25 minutes.
3. Serve once cooled.

Nutritional Facts (Per Serving): Calories: 225 | Protein: 8g | Fat: 5g | Carbs: 26g | Fiber: 2g | Sodium: 310mg | Sugars: 7g

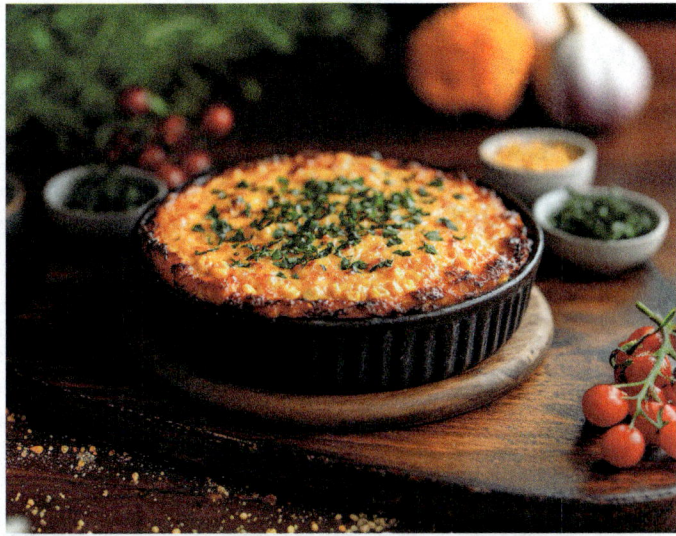

Low-acid cornbread with cheese

Prep: 10 minutes | Cook: 25 minutes | Serves:2

Ingredients:

- 1/2 cup whole wheat flour (60g)
- 1/2 cup cornmeal (60g)
- 1/4 cup shredded low-fat cheddar cheese (30g)
- 1/4 cup corn kernels (40g)
- 1/2 tsp baking powder (2g)
- 1/4 cup almond milk (60ml)
- 1 tbsp olive oil (15ml)

Instructions:

1. Preheat oven to 375°F (190°C). Mix flour, cornmeal, baking powder, and olive oil.
2. Add almond milk, cheese, and corn kernels, stirring until combined.
3. Pour into a greased baking dish and bake for 20-25 minutes until golden.

Nutritional Facts (Per Serving): Calories: 211 | Protein: 8g | Fat: 6g | Carbs: 24g | Fiber: 2g | Sodium: 330mg | Sugars: 5g

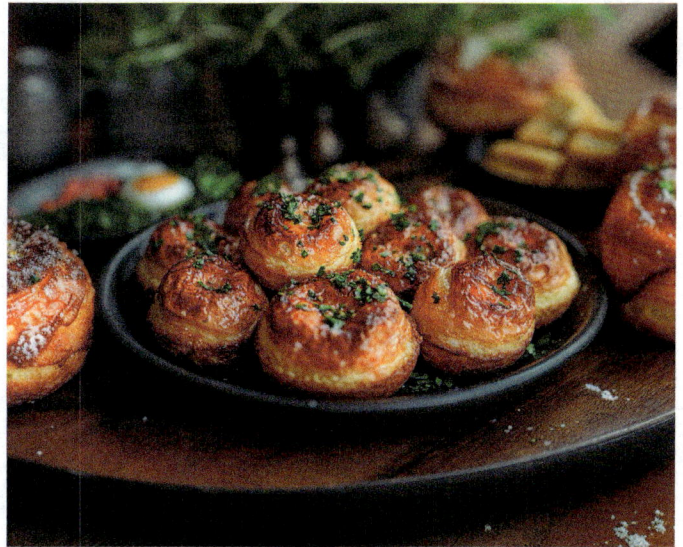

Low-acid American popovers

Prep: 10 minutes | Cook: 20 minutes | Serves:2

Ingredients:

- 1/2 cup whole wheat flour (60g)
- 1/4 tsp salt (1g)
- 1 egg (50g)
- 1/2 cup almond milk (120ml)
- 1 tsp olive oil (5ml)

Instructions:

1. Preheat oven to 425°F (220°C) and grease a muffin tin with olive oil.
2. Whisk together flour, salt, egg, and almond milk until smooth.
3. Pour the batter into the muffin tin and bake for 15-20 minutes until puffed and golden.

Nutritional Facts (Per Serving): Calories: 216 | Protein: 9g | Fat: 5g | Carbs: 24g | Fiber: 1g | Sodium: 320mg | Sugars: 4g

CHAPTER 16: DINNER: Gentle and nourishing evening salads

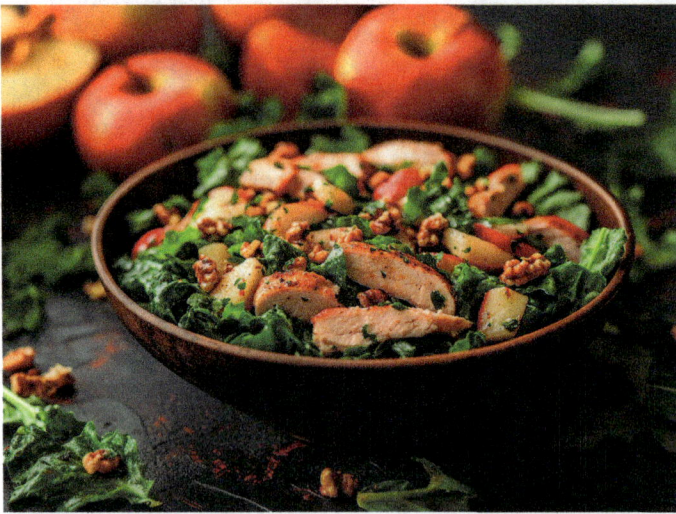

Turkey and apple walnut salad

Prep: 10 minutes | Cook: 0 minutes | Serves: 1

Ingredients:

- 2 cups mixed greens (60g)
- 3 oz sliced turkey breast (85g)
- 1/2 apple, sliced (75g)
- 1 tbsp chopped walnuts (15g)
- 1 tbsp honey mustard dressing (15ml)

Instructions:

1. Toss mixed greens with turkey slices, apple, and walnuts in a large bowl.
2. Drizzle honey mustard dressing on top and gently mix.
3. Serve immediately.

Nutritional Facts (Per Serving): Calories: 367 | Protein: 16g | Fat: 12g | Carbs: 43g | Fiber: 7g | Sodium: 450mg | Sugars: 9g

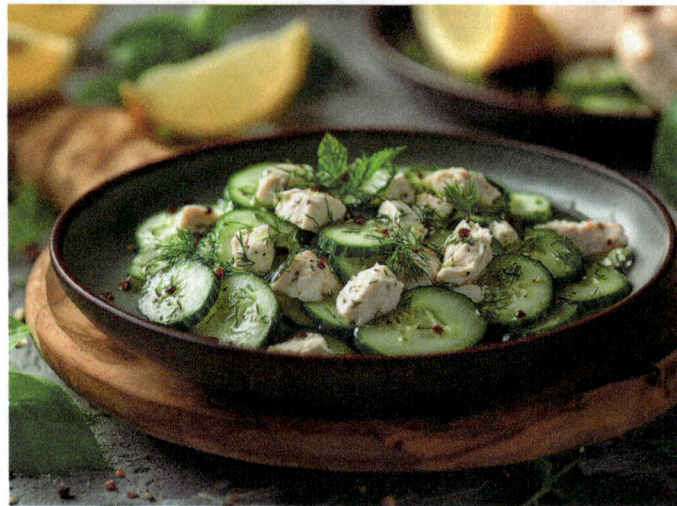

Cucumber and dill yogurt salad

Prep: 10 minutes | Cook: 10 minutes | Serves:1

Ingredients:

- 1 cup sliced cucumber (120g)
- 3 oz boiled chicken breast, shredded (85g)
- 1/4 cup Greek yogurt (60g)
- 1 tbsp fresh dill, chopped (5g)
- 1/2 tsp lemon juice (2ml)

Instructions:

1. Combine sliced cucumber, shredded chicken, and dill in a bowl.
2. Add Greek yogurt and lemon juice, and mix until well coated.
3. Serve chilled.

Nutritional Information (Per Serving): Calories: 380 | Protein: 18g | Fat: 11g | Carbs: 41g | Fiber: 6g | Sodium: 440mg | Sugars: 7g

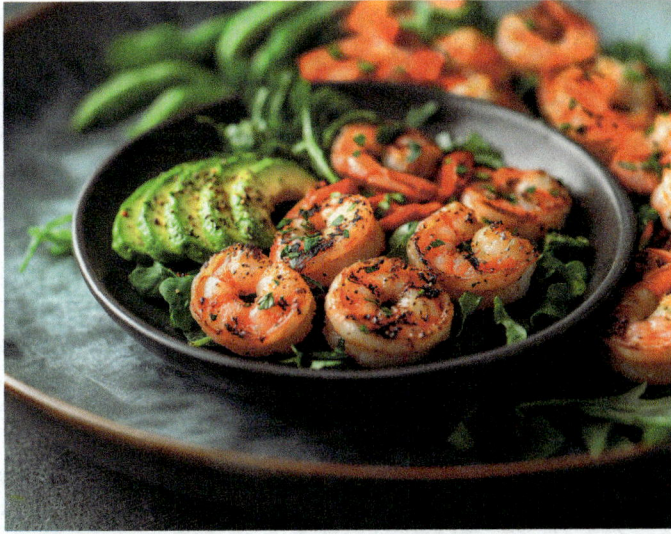

Shrimp and avocado salad

Prep: 15 minutes | Cook: 5 minutes | Serves: 1

Ingredients:

- 2 cups mixed greens (60g)
- 3 oz grilled shrimp (85g)
- 1/2 avocado, sliced (70g)
- 1/4 cup steamed asparagus (50g)
- 2 tbsp Greek yogurt dressing (30g)

Instructions:

1. Place mixed greens on a plate and top with grilled shrimp, avocado slices, and steamed asparagus.
2. Drizzle Greek yogurt dressing over the salad.
3. Serve fresh.

Nutritional Facts (Per Serving): Calories: 378 | Protein: 17g | Fat: 12g | Carbs: 42g | Fiber: 7g | Sodium: 450mg | Sugars: 6g

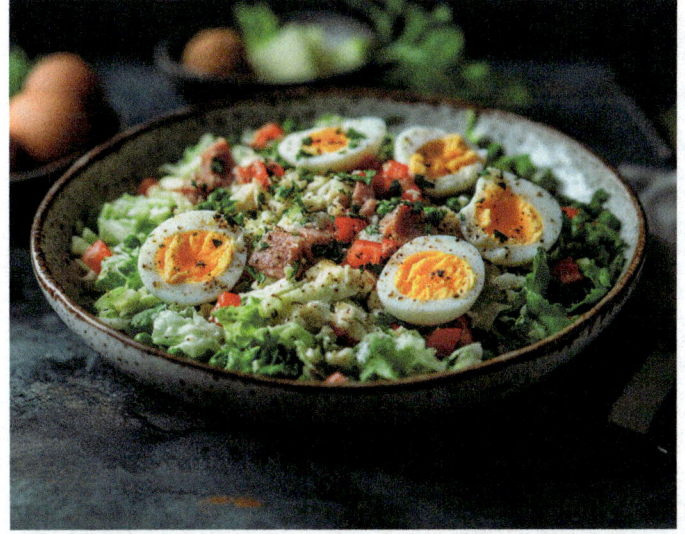

Welsh salad without peas

Prep: 15 minutes | Cook: 10 minutes | Serves: 2

Ingredients:

- 4 oz boiled lean meat, sliced (115g)
- 2 cups shredded white cabbage (120g)
- 1 medium apple, diced (150g)
- 1/4 cup shredded cheese (30g)
- 4 quail eggs, hard-boiled and halved (40g)
- 1/4 cup plain yogurt (60g)
- Salt to taste (1g)

Instructions:

1. In a large bowl, combine sliced meat, shredded cabbage, diced apple, and shredded cheese.
2. Add the halved quail eggs on top.
3. Drizzle with plain yogurt and season with salt.
4. Toss gently to combine and serve immediately.

Nutritional Facts (Per Serving): Calories: 382 | Protein: 18g | Fat: 14g | Carbs: 28g | Fiber: 8g | Sodium: 450mg | Sugars: 7g

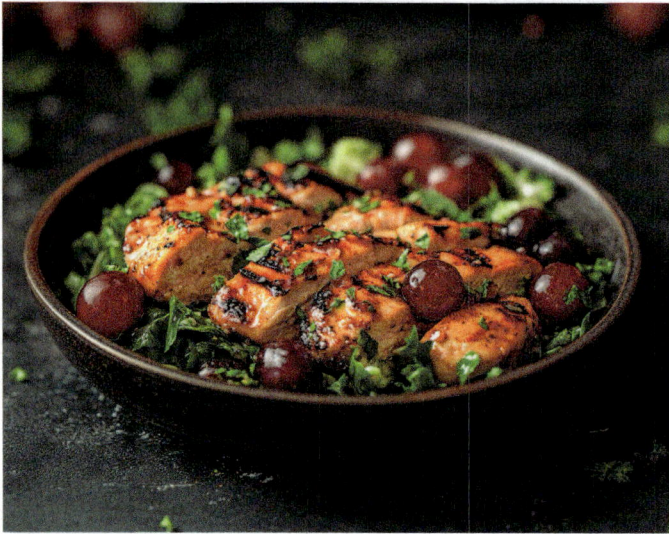

Chicken and grape salad

Prep: 10 minutes | Cook: 10 minutes | Serves: 2

Ingredients:

- 2 cups mixed greens (60g)
- 4 oz grilled chicken breast, sliced (115g)
- 1/2 cup red grapes, halved (75g)
- 1/4 cup plain Greek yogurt (60g)
- 1 tbsp apple cider vinegar (15ml)
- 1 tbsp olive oil (15ml)
- Salt to taste (1g)

Instructions:

1. In a large bowl, combine mixed greens, sliced grilled chicken, and halved grapes.
2. In a small bowl, whisk together Greek yogurt, apple cider vinegar, olive oil, and salt.
3. Drizzle the yogurt dressing over the salad and toss to combine. Serve chilled.

Nutritional Facts (Per Serving): Calories: 386 | Protein: 19g | Fat: 14g | Carbs: 25g | Fiber: 7g | Sodium: 430mg | Sugars: 7g

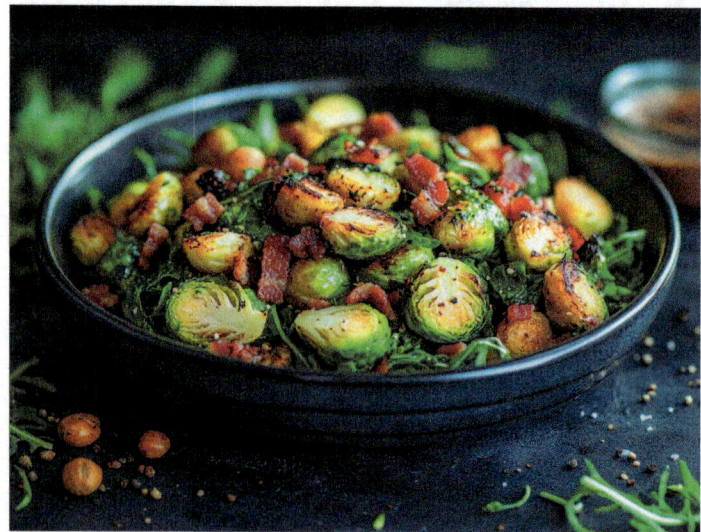

Warm brussels sprouts and bacon salad

Prep: 10 minutes | Cook: 20 minutes | Serves: 2

Ingredients:

- 2 cups brussels sprouts, halved (160g)
- 2 slices turkey bacon, chopped (30g)
- 2 cups mixed greens (60g)
- 1 tbsp olive oil (15ml)
- 1 tbsp whole grain mustard (15g)
- 1 tbsp apple cider vinegar (15ml)
- Salt and allspice to taste (1g each)

Instructions:

1. Preheat oven to 400°F (200°C). Toss brussels sprouts with olive oil, salt, and allspice.
2. Roast for 20 minutes until tender.
3. Cook turkey bacon in a skillet until crispy.
4. In a large bowl, combine roasted brussels sprouts, cooked bacon, and mixed greens.
5. In a small bowl, whisk together mustard and apple cider vinegar.
6. Drizzle the mustard vinaigrette over the salad and toss to combine. Serve warm.

Nutritional Facts (Per Serving): Calories: 365 | Protein: 18g | Fat: 15g | Carbs: 22g | Fiber: 8g | Sodium: 450mg | Sugars: 7g

CHAPTER 17: DINNER: Wholesome veggie delights for dinner

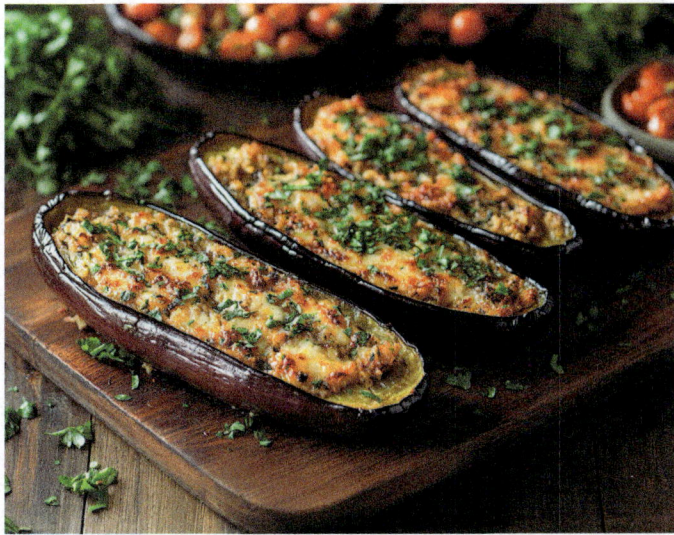

Stuffed eggplants baked with cheese crust

Prep: 15 minutes | Cook: 30 minutes | Serves: 2

Ingredients:

- 1 medium eggplant, halved (300g)
- 1/2 cup low-fat ricotta cheese (120g)
- 1/4 cup grated parmesan cheese (30g)
- 1/4 cup diced tomatoes (60g)
- 1 tbsp olive oil (15ml)
- 1 garlic clove, minced (2g)
- 1 tsp dried oregano (1g)
- Salt and allspice to taste

Instructions:

1. Preheat oven to 375°F (190°C).
2. Scoop out the flesh of the eggplant halves, leaving a 1/2-inch shell. Chop the flesh.
3. Sauté the chopped eggplant, garlic, and diced tomatoes in olive oil for 5 minutes.
4. Mix in ricotta cheese, oregano, salt, and allspice.
5. Stuff the eggplant shells with the mixture, top with grated parmesan.
6. Bake for 25-30 minutes until golden brown.

Nutritional Facts (Per Serving): Calories: 367 | Protein: 17g | Fat: 14g | Carbs: 24g | Fiber: 8g | Sodium: 450mg | Sugars: 7g

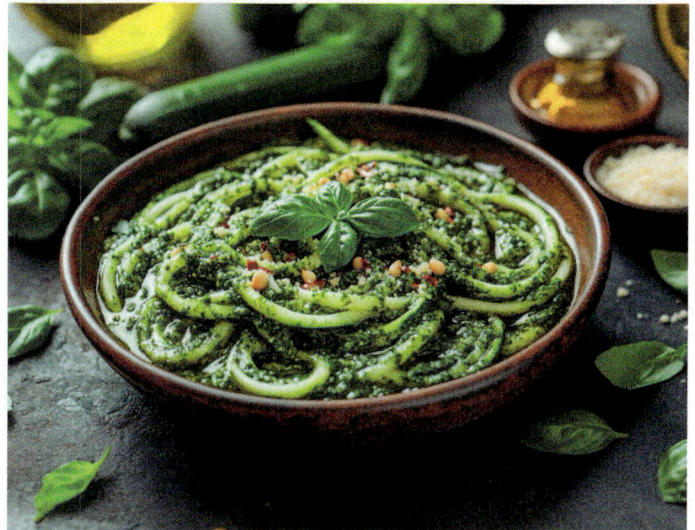

Zucchini noodles with pesto

Prep: 10 minutes | Cook: 5 minutes | Serves: 2

Ingredients:

- 2 medium zucchinis, spiralized (300g)
- 1/4 cup fresh basil leaves (10g)
- 1 tbsp pine nuts (15g)
- 1 garlic clove (2g)
- 1/4 cup olive oil (60ml)
- 2 tbsp grated parmesan cheese (30g)
- Salt and allspice to taste

Instructions:

1. In a food processor, blend basil, pine nuts, garlic, and olive oil until smooth.
2. Toss the zucchini noodles with the pesto.
3. Sprinkle with grated parmesan, season with salt and allspice.
4. Serve immediately.

Nutritional Facts (Per Serving): Calories: 372 | Protein: 15g | Fat: 15g | Carbs: 16g | Fiber: 7g | Sodium: 400mg | Sugars: 6g

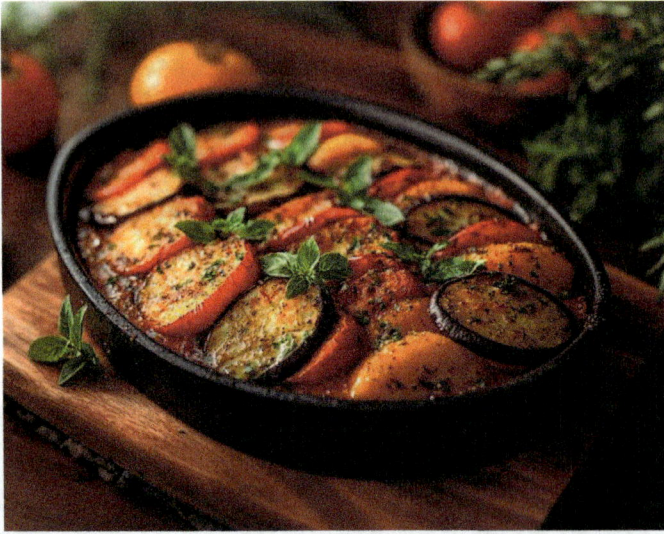

Eggplant and bell peppers bake

Prep:10 minutes | Cook: 30 minutes | Serves: 2

Ingredients:

- 1 medium eggplant, sliced (300g)
- 1 red bell pepper, sliced (150g)
- 1 yellow bell pepper, sliced (150g)
- 1/2 cup marinara sauce (120g)
- 1/4 cup grated parmesan cheese (30g)
- 1 tbsp olive oil (15ml)
- Salt and allspice to taste

Instructions:

1. Preheat oven to 375°F (190°C).
2. Layer the eggplant and bell pepper slices in a baking dish.
3. Drizzle with olive oil and top with marinara sauce.
4. Sprinkle with parmesan cheese, season with salt and allspice.
5. Bake for 30 minutes until vegetables are tender and cheese is golden.

Nutritional Facts (Per Serving): Calories: 365 | Protein: 16g | Fat: 14g | Carbs: 24g | Fiber: 8g | Sodium: 450mg | Sugars: 7g

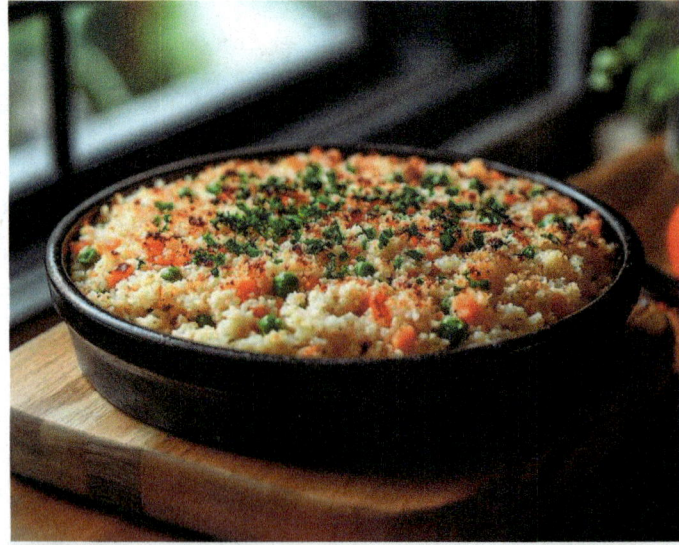

Cauliflower rice bake

Prep: 10 minutes | Cook: 20 minutes | Serves: 2

Ingredients:

- 2 cups cauliflower rice (240g)
- 1/2 cup mixed vegetables (carrots, peas) (60g)
- 1 tbsp soy sauce (15ml)
- 1 tbsp olive oil (15ml)
- 1 garlic clove, minced (2g)
- 1/4 cup grated parmesan cheese (30g)
- Salt and allspice to taste

Instructions:

1. Preheat oven to 375°F (190°C).
2. Sauté cauliflower rice and mixed vegetables in olive oil for 5 minutes.
3. Stir in soy sauce and garlic.
4. Transfer to a baking dish, top with parmesan cheese.
5. Bake for 15 minutes until cheese is golden.

Nutritional Facts (Per Serving): Calories: 370 | Protein: 16g | Fat: 14g | Carbs: 20g | Fiber: 7g | Sodium: 450mg | Sugars: 7g

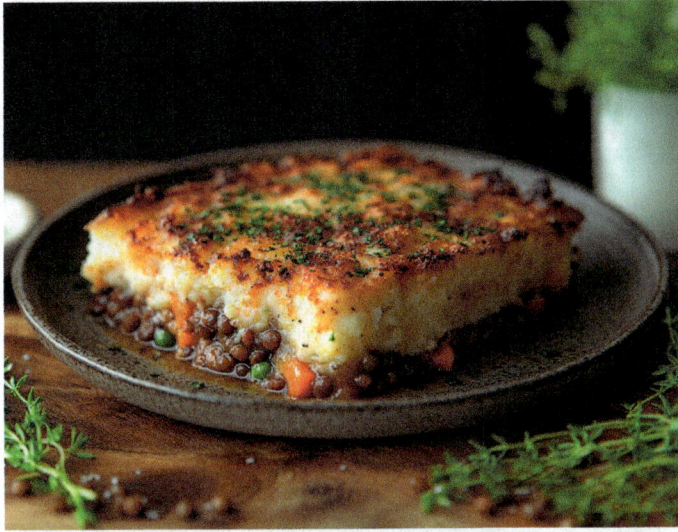

Cauliflower and lentil shepherd's pie

Prep: 15 minutes | Cook: 35 minutes | Serves: 2

Ingredients:

- 1 cup cooked lentils (150g)
- 2 cups mashed cauliflower (240g)
- 1/2 cup mixed vegetables (carrots, peas) (60g)
- 1 garlic clove, minced (2g)
- 1 tbsp olive oil (15ml)
- 1 tbsp low-carb sweetener (12g)
- 1/4 cup grated parmesan cheese (30g)
- Salt and allspice to taste

Instructions:

1. Preheat oven to 375°F (190°C).
2. Sauté mixed vegetables and garlic in olive oil for 5 minutes.
3. Stir in cooked lentils and season with salt and allspice.
4. Transfer mixture to a baking dish, top with mashed cauliflower.
5. Sprinkle with parmesan cheese.
6. Bake for 25 minutes until golden brown.

Nutritional Facts (Per Serving): Calories: 376 | Protein: 17g | Fat: 14g | Carbs: 26g | Fiber: 8g | Sodium: 450mg | Sugars: 7g

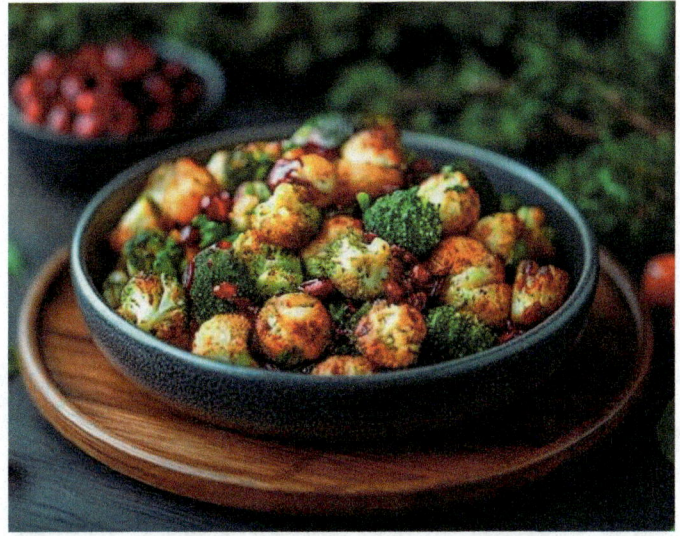

Roasted brussels sprouts with balsamic glaze

Prep: 10 minutes | Cook: 25 minutes | Serves: 2

Ingredients:

- 2 cups a mix of broccoli, brussels sprouts and mashed cauliflower, halved (300g)
- 1 tbsp olive oil (15ml)
- 1 tbsp honey (15g)
- 2 tbsp balsamic vinegar (30ml)
- Salt and allspice to taste

Instructions:

1. Preheat oven to 400°F (200°C).
2. Toss cabbage mix with olive oil, salt, and allspice.
3. Roast for 20 minutes until crispy.
4. Drizzle with balsamic vinegar and honey, roast for an additional 5 minutes.
5. Serve warm.

Nutritional Facts (Per Serving): Calories: 374 | Protein: 16g | Fat: 14g | Carbs: 28g | Fiber: 8g | Sodium: 450mg | Sugars: 8g

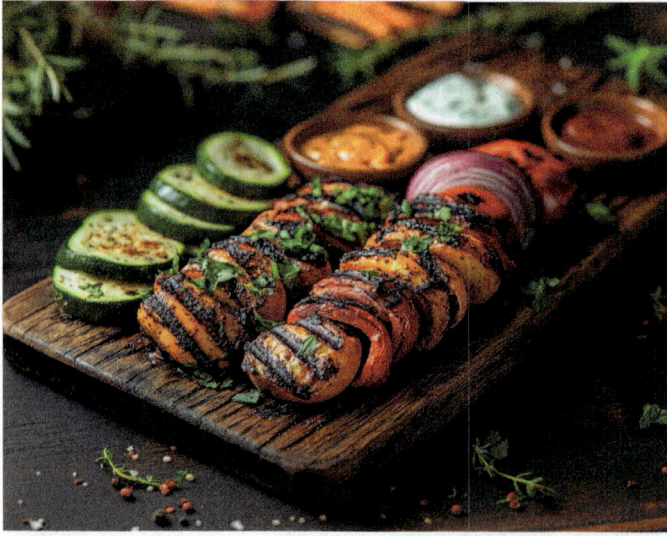

Grilled vegetable fajitas with cashew cheese sauce

Prep:15 minutes | Cook: 20 minutes | Serves: 2

Ingredients:

- 1 red bell pepper, sliced (150g)
- 1 green bell pepper, sliced (150g)
- 1 small zucchini, sliced (150g)
- 1 small onion, sliced (100g)
- 1 tbsp olive oil (15ml)
- 1/2 cup cashews, soaked and drained (60g)
- 1/4 cup water (60ml)
- 1 tbsp apple cider vinegar (15ml)
- 1 tbsp nutritional yeast (15g)
- Salt and allspice to taste

Instructions:

1. Preheat grill to medium heat.
2. Toss bell peppers, zucchini, and onion with olive oil, salt, and allspice.
3. Grill vegetables for 10-15 minutes until tender.
4. In a blender, blend cashews, water, apple cider vinegar, and nutritional yeast until smooth.
5. Serve grilled vegetables drizzled with cashew cheese sauce.

Nutritional Facts (Per Serving): Calories: 373 | Protein: 16g | Fat: 14g | Carbs: 28g | Fiber: 8g | Sodium: 450mg | Sugars: 8g

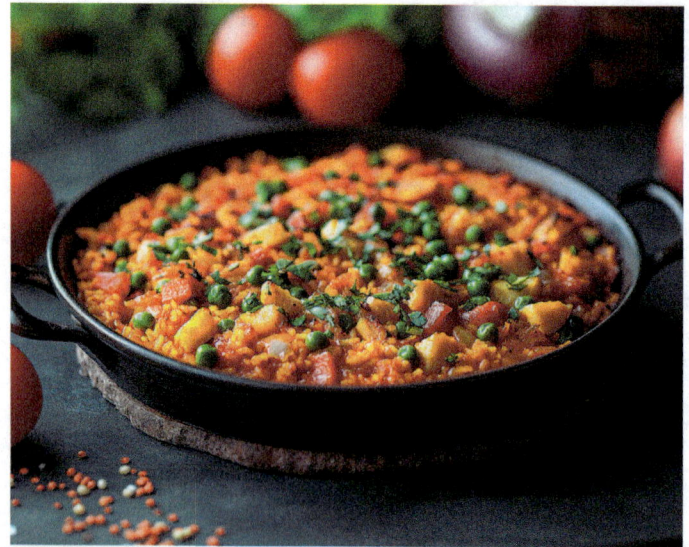

Vegetable paella

Prep: 15 minutes | Cook: 25 minutes | Serves: 2

Ingredients:

- 1 cup cauliflower rice (120g)
- 1/2 cup mixed vegetables (peas, carrots, green beans) (60g)
- 1 small onion, chopped (100g)
- 1 garlic clove, minced (2g)
- 1 tbsp olive oil (15ml)
- 1/2 tsp smoked paprika (2g)
- 1/4 tsp saffron threads (1g)
- 1/4 cup vegetable broth (60ml)
- Salt and allspice to taste

Instructions:

1. Heat olive oil in a large pan over medium heat.
2. Sauté onion, garlic, and mixed vegetables for 5 minutes.
3. Stir in cauliflower rice, paprika, saffron, vegetable broth, salt, and allspice.
4. Cook for 10-15 minutes until vegetables are tender and broth is absorbed. Serve hot.

Nutritional Facts (Per Serving): Calories: 363 | Protein: 16g | Fat: 14g | Carbs: 24g | Fiber: 8g | Sodium: 450mg | Sugars: 8g

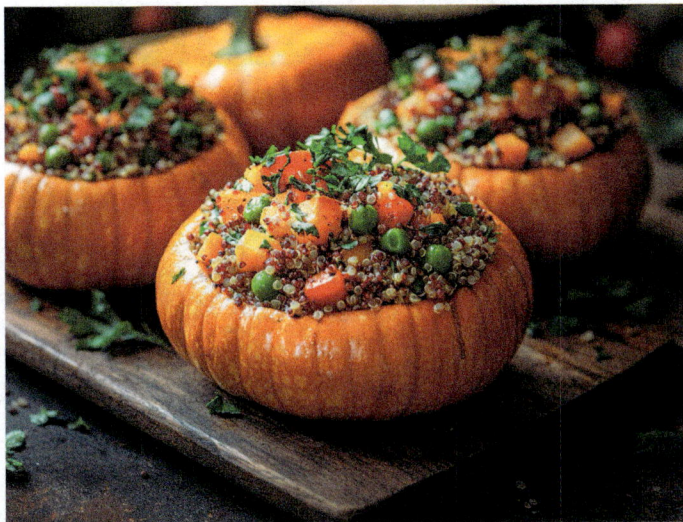

Mini pumpkins stuffed with mixed vegetables and cheese

Prep: 15 minutes | Cook: 30 minutes | Serves: 2

Ingredients:

- 2 mini pumpkins (400g)
- 1/2 cup quinoa, cooked (90g)
- 1/4 cup low-fat cheddar cheese, shredded (30g)
- 1/2 cup mixed vegetables (carrots, peas, bell peppers) (60g)
- 1 tbsp olive oil (15ml)
- Salt and allspice to taste

Instructions:

1. Preheat oven to 375°F (190°C).
2. Cut tops off pumpkins, scoop out seeds.
3. Toss mixed vegetables with cooked quinoa, olive oil, salt, and allspice.
4. Stuff pumpkins with the mixture, top with shredded cheese.
5. Place pumpkins in a baking dish, bake for 25-30 minutes until tender.

Nutritional Facts (Per Serving): Calories: 367 | Protein: 16g | Fat: 14g | Carbs: 28g | Fiber: 8g | Sodium: 450mg | Sugars: 8g

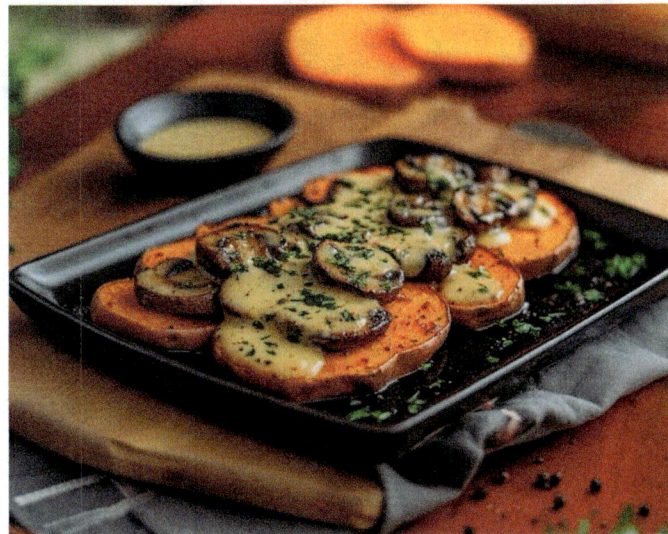

Sweet potatoes and mushrooms with cheese sauce

Prep: 15 minutes | Cook: 25 minutes | Serves: 2

Ingredients:

- 1 medium sweet potato, sliced (200g)
- 1 cup mushrooms, sliced (120g)
- 1/2 cup low-fat cheddar cheese, shredded (60g)
- 1/4 cup milk (60ml)
- 1 tbsp olive oil (15ml)
- 1 garlic clove, minced (2g)
- Salt and allspice to taste

Instructions:

1. Preheat oven to 375°F (190°C).
2. Sauté mushrooms and garlic in olive oil for 5 minutes.
3. Layer sweet potato slices in a baking dish, top with sautéed mushrooms.
4. In a small pot, heat milk and cheese until melted, pour over vegetables.
5. Bake for 20-25 minutes until sweet potatoes are tender.

Nutritional Facts (Per Serving): Calories: 376 | Protein: 16g | Fat: 14g | Carbs: 28g | Fiber: 8g | Sodium: 450mg | Sugars: 8g

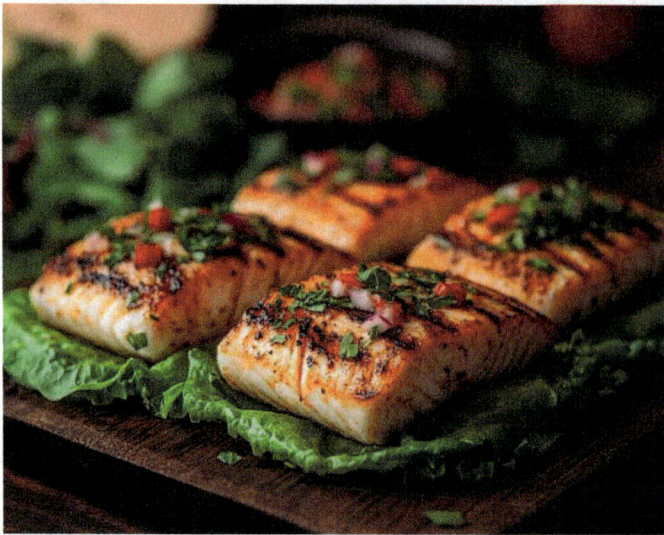

Fish lettuce wraps with cabbage slaw

Prep: 15 minutes | Cook: 10 minutes | Serves: 2

Ingredients:

- 6 oz grilled white fish (170g)
- 4 large lettuce leaves (60g)
- 1 cup shredded cabbage (80g)
- 2 tbsp plain Greek yogurt (30g)
- 1 tsp apple cider vinegar (5ml)
- 1 tbsp olive oil (15ml)
- Salt and allspice to taste

Instructions:

1. Grill the fish over medium heat for 4-5 minutes on each side until fully cooked.
2. In a bowl, mix shredded cabbage with Greek yogurt, apple cider vinegar, olive oil, salt, and allspice to make the slaw.
3. Place the grilled fish in the lettuce leaves and top with the cabbage slaw. Serve immediately.

Nutritional Facts (Per Serving): Calories: 375 | Protein: 20g | Fat: 14g | Carbs: 12g | Fiber: 7g | Sodium: 420mg | Sugars: 7g

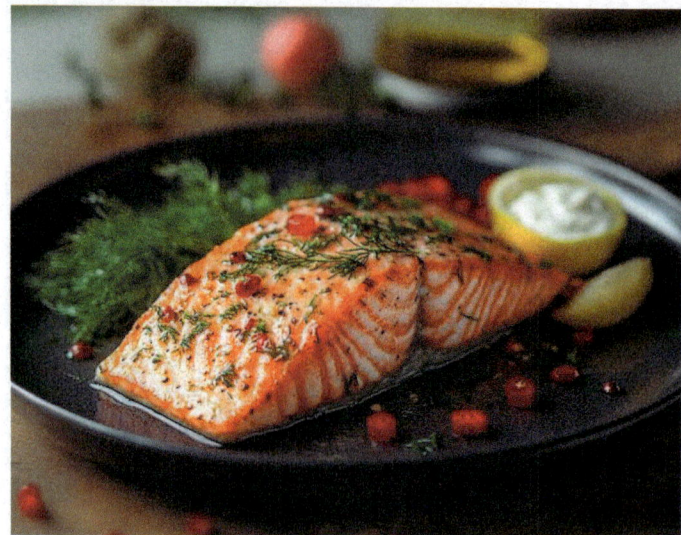

Poached salmon with dill sauce

Prep: 10 minutes | Cook: 40 minutes | Serves: 2

Ingredients:

- 2 salmon fillets (6 oz each) (170g each)
- 2 cups water (480ml)
- 1 tbsp fresh dill, chopped (15g)
- 2 tbsp plain Greek yogurt (30g)
- 1 tsp apple cider vinegar (5ml)
- 1 tsp olive oil (5ml)
- Salt and allspice to taste

Instructions:

1. Bring water to a simmer in a deep pan. Add salmon fillets and poach for 10-12 minutes until fully cooked.
2. In a small bowl, mix Greek yogurt, fresh dill, apple cider vinegar, olive oil, salt, and allspice to make the dill sauce.
3. Serve the poached salmon with the dill sauce on top.

Nutritional Facts (Per Serving): Calories: 369 | Protein: 20g | Fat: 15g | Carbs: 6g | Fiber: 7g | Sodium: 450mg | Sugars: 6g

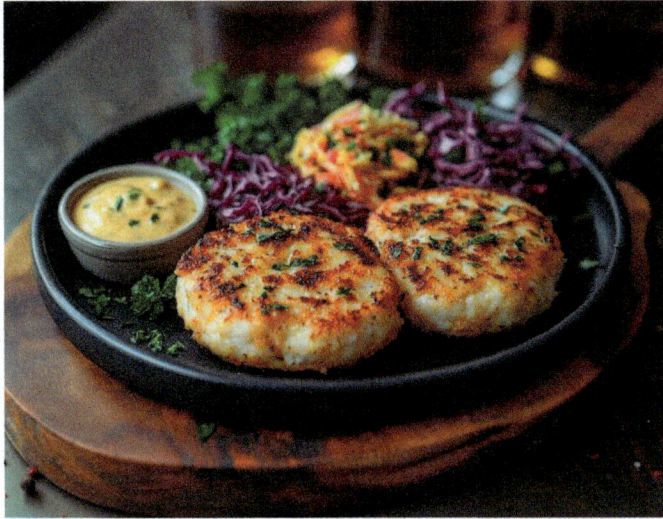

Haddock cutlets with cabbage salad and cheese sauce

Prep: 15 minutes | Cook: 20 minutes | Serves: 2

Ingredients:

- 8 oz haddock fillets (225g)
- 1/2 cup whole wheat breadcrumbs (60g)
- 1 egg white (30g)
- 2 cups shredded cabbage (160g)
- 2 tbsp plain Greek yogurt (30g)
- 1/4 cup shredded low-fat cheddar cheese (30g)
- 1 tsp olive oil (5ml)
- Salt and allspice to taste

Instructions:

1. Preheat oven to 375°F (190°C). Mix haddock fillets with egg white and breadcrumbs to form cutlets. Bake for 15-20 minutes.
2. In a bowl, mix shredded cabbage with Greek yogurt, salt, and allspice to make the salad.
3. Melt the cheddar cheese with a little water over low heat to create a cheese sauce.
4. Serve the haddock cutlets with cabbage salad and drizzle with cheese sauce.

Nutritional Facts (Per Serving): Calories: 367 | Protein: 20g | Fat: 14g | Carbs: 20g | Fiber: 7g | Sodium: 450mg | Sugars: 7g

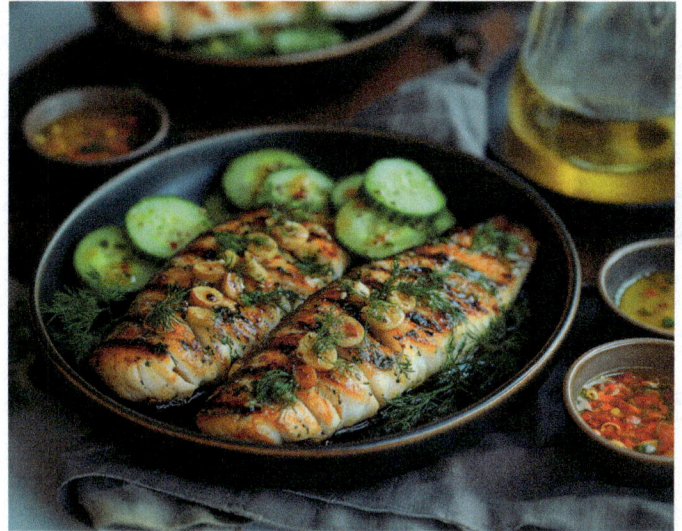

Grilled mackerel with cucumber salad

Prep: 15 minutes | Cook: 10 minutes | Serves: 2

Ingredients:

- 2 mackerel fillets (6 oz each) (170g each)
- 1 cucumber, sliced (150g)
- 1 tbsp fresh dill, chopped (15g)
- 2 tbsp plain Greek yogurt (30g)
- 1 tsp apple cider vinegar (5ml)
- 1 tbsp olive oil (15ml)
- Salt and allspice to taste

Instructions:

1. Marinate the mackerel fillets in apple cider vinegar, salt, and allspice for 10 minutes. Grill over medium heat for 4-5 minutes per side.
2. In a bowl, mix cucumber slices, fresh dill, Greek yogurt, olive oil, salt, and allspice to make the cucumber salad.
3. Serve the grilled mackerel with the cucumber salad on the side.

Nutritional Facts (Per Serving): Calories: 354 | Protein: 20g | Fat: 14g | Carbs: 10g | Fiber: 7g | Sodium: 420mg | Sugars: 7g

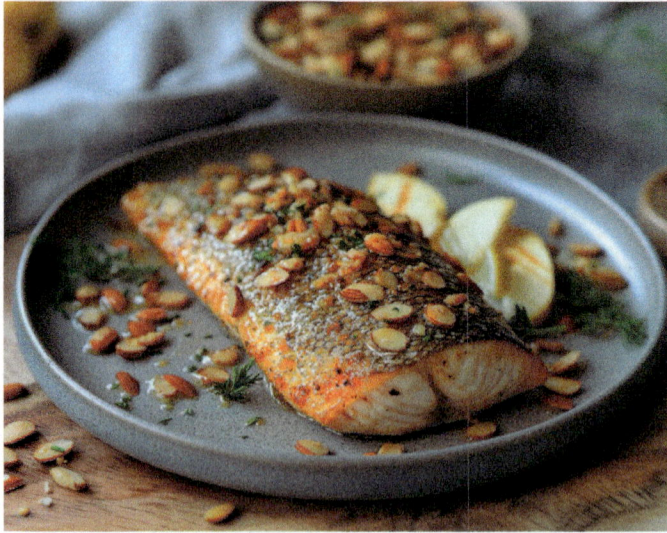

Baked trout with almonds

Prep: 10 minutes | Cook: 20 minutes | Serves: 2

Ingredients:

- 2 trout fillets (6 oz each) (170g each)
- 2 tbsp sliced almonds (30g)
- 1 tbsp olive oil (15ml)
- 1 tsp apple cider vinegar (5ml)
- Salt and allspice to taste

Instructions:

1. Preheat oven to 375°F (190°C). Place the trout fillets on a baking sheet, drizzle with olive oil, and season with salt, allspice, and apple cider vinegar.
2. Sprinkle sliced almonds on top of the trout fillets.
3. Bake for 15-20 minutes or until the trout is fully cooked and the almonds are golden brown.
4. Serve immediately.

Nutritional Facts (Per Serving): Calories: 376 | Protein: 20g | Fat: 14g | Carbs: 6g | Fiber: 7g | Sodium: 400mg | Sugars: 6g

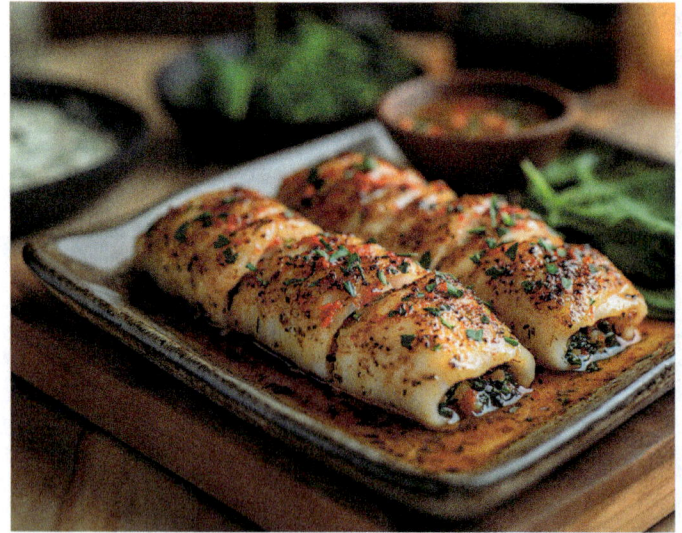

Stuffed calamari with spinach-lemon dressing

Prep: 20 minutes | Cook: 25 minutes | Serves: 2

Ingredients:

- 4 large calamari tubes (10 oz total) (280g)
- 1/2 cup diced mixed vegetables (carrot, celery) (80g)
- 1 tsp apple cider vinegar (5ml)
- 2 tbsp olive oil (30ml)
- 1/2 cup cooked brown rice (80g)
- 2 cups fresh spinach (60g)
- Salt and allspice to taste

Instructions:

1. Preheat oven to 350°F (175°C). In a bowl, mix cooked brown rice and diced vegetables. Stuff the calamari tubes with the mixture and secure with toothpicks.
2. Place the stuffed calamari in a baking dish, drizzle with 1 tbsp olive oil, and bake for 20 minutes.
3. In a skillet, sauté the spinach in the remaining olive oil and apple cider vinegar until wilted. Season with salt and allspice.
4. Serve the stuffed calamari over the sautéed spinach.

Nutritional Facts (Per Serving): Calories: 376 | Protein: 18g | Fat: 15g | Carbs: 22g | Fiber: 8g | Sodium: 430mg | Sugars: 7g

CHAPTER 19 DINNER: Celebratory and family-friendly meals without discomfort

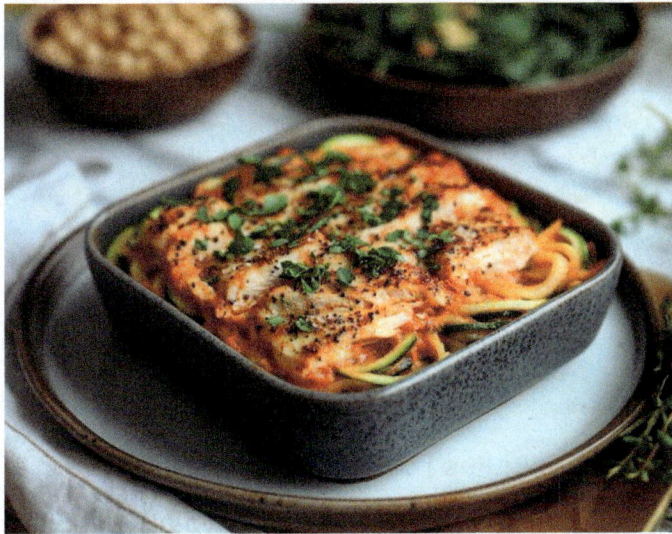

Chicken and spinach zucchini noodle bake

Prep: 15 minutes | Cook: 25 minutes | Serves: 2

Ingredients:

- 2 medium zucchini, spiralized (300g)
- 1 chicken breast, cooked and shredded (200g)
- 2 cups fresh spinach (60g)
- 1/2 cup low-fat mozzarella cheese, shredded (60g)
- 1/4 cup unsweetened almond milk (60ml)
- 1 tbsp olive oil (15ml)
- 1/4 tsp garlic powder (1g)
- Salt and allspice to taste

Instructions:

1. Preheat the oven to 375°F (190°C).
2. In a pan, heat olive oil over medium heat and sauté spinach until wilted.
3. Combine zucchini noodles, shredded chicken, sautéed spinach, almond milk, garlic powder, salt, and allspice in a mixing bowl.
4. Transfer the mixture to a baking dish, sprinkle with shredded mozzarella, and bake for 20 minutes, until cheese is melted and bubbly.

Nutritional Facts (Per Serving): Calories: 365 | Protein: 18g | Fat: 13g | Carbs: 15g | Fiber: 8g | Sodium: 450mg | Sugars: 7g

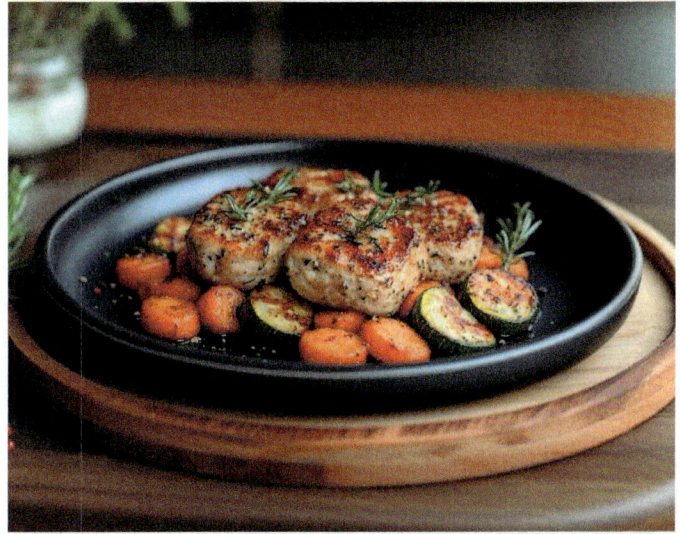

Turkey cutlets with roasted vegetables

Prep: 10 minutes | Cook: 25 minutes | Serves: 2

Ingredients:

- 1/2 lb ground turkey (225g)
- 1/2 tsp onion powder (2g)
- 1/2 tsp garlic powder (2g)
- 1 tbsp olive oil (15ml)
- 1 medium carrot, chopped (100g)
- 1 medium zucchini, chopped (150g)
- Salt and allspice to taste

Instructions:

1. Preheat the oven to 400°F (200°C).
2. In a bowl, mix ground turkey with onion powder, garlic powder, salt, and allspice. Form into cutlets.
3. Heat olive oil in a pan over medium heat and sear the cutlets until browned on both sides.
4. Arrange cutlets, carrots, and zucchini on a baking sheet, drizzle with remaining olive oil, and roast for 15-20 minutes, until vegetables are tender and cutlets are fully cooked.

Nutritional Facts (Per Serving): Calories: 369 | Protein: 20g | Fat: 14g | Carbs: 18g | Fiber: 7g | Sodium: 450mg | Sugars: 6g

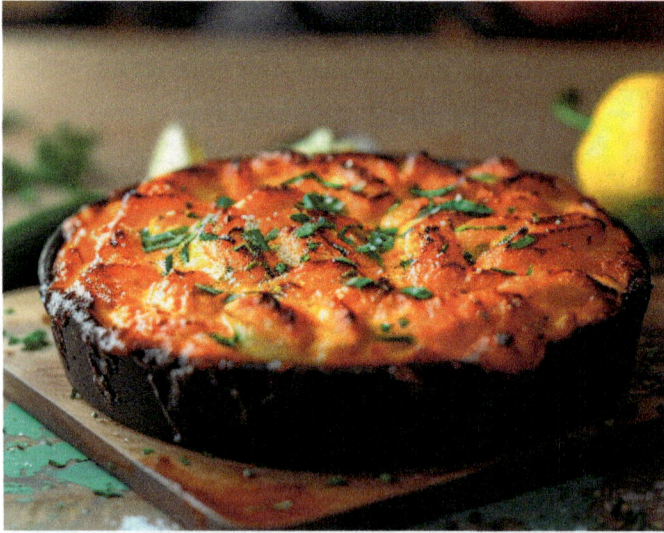

Chicken and mushroom casserole

Prep: 15 minutes | Cook: 30 minutes | Serves: 2

Ingredients:

- 1 chicken breast, diced (200g)
- 1 cup mushrooms, sliced (100g)
- 1/2 cup low-fat mozzarella cheese, shredded (60g)
- 1/4 cup unsweetened almond milk (60ml)
- 1 tbsp olive oil (15ml)
- 1/2 tsp thyme (1g)
- Salt and allspice to taste

Instructions:

1. Preheat the oven to 375°F (190°C).
2. Heat olive oil in a pan over medium heat, sauté mushrooms until tender, then add diced chicken and cook until no longer pink.
3. In a baking dish, combine cooked chicken and mushrooms, almond milk, thyme, salt, and allspice.
4. Top with shredded mozzarella.
5. Bake for 25-30 minutes, until cheese is melted and golden.

Nutritional Facts (Per Serving): Calories: 374 | Protein: 19g | Fat: 13.5g | Carbs: 14g | Fiber: 7g | Sodium: 400mg | Sugars: 7g

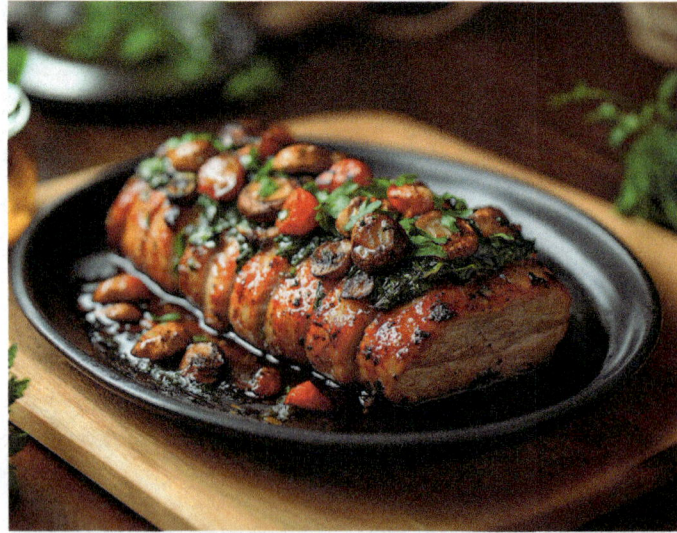

Stuffed pork tenderloin

Prep: 20 minutes | Cook: 35 minutes | Serves: 2

Ingredients:

- 1 pork tenderloin, butterflied (300g)
- 1 cup fresh spinach (30g)
- 1/2 cup mushrooms, diced (50g)
- 1/4 cup low-fat mozzarella cheese, shredded (30g)
- 1 tbsp olive oil (15ml)
- 1/2 tsp garlic powder (2g)
- Salt and allspice to taste

Instructions:

1. Preheat the oven to 375°F (190°C).
2. In a pan, heat olive oil over medium heat, sauté spinach and mushrooms until tender.
3. Lay the butterflied pork tenderloin flat, season with garlic powder, salt, and allspice, and spread the spinach-mushroom mixture evenly over the pork.
4. Sprinkle with cheese and roll up tightly, securing with kitchen twine.
5. Place the stuffed tenderloin in a baking dish and bake for 25-30 minutes, until cooked through.

Nutritional Facts (Per Serving): Calories: 379 | Protein: 20g | Fat: 14g | Carbs: 10g | Fiber: 7g | Sodium: 450mg | Sugars: 6g

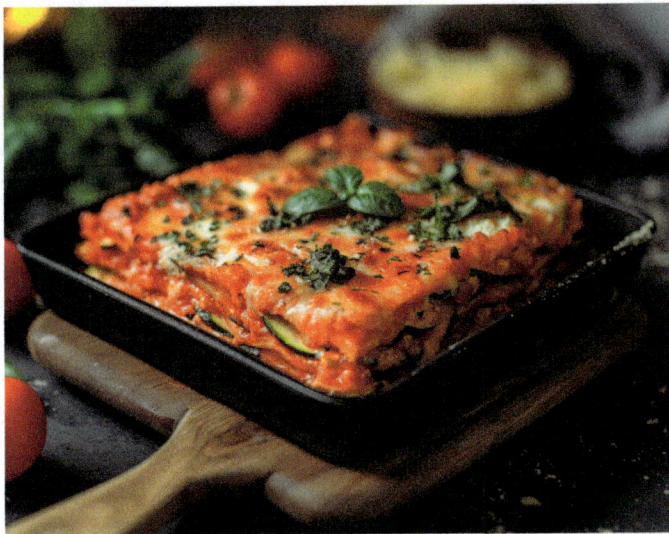

Vegetable lasagna with zucchini noodles

Prep: 20 minutes | Cook: 30 minutes | Serves: 2

Ingredients:

- 2 medium zucchini, sliced into thin strips (300g)
- 1 cup ricotta cheese (120g)
- 1 cup fresh spinach (30g)
- 1/2 tsp Italian seasoning (2g)
- 1/2 cup low-fat mozzarella cheese, shredded (60g)
- 1/4 cup grated Parmesan cheese (30g)
- 1 tbsp olive oil (15ml)
- Salt and allspice to taste

Sauce:
- 2 large red bell peppers (300g)
- 1 small onion, chopped (50g)
- 2 tbsp olive oil (30ml)
- 1/4 cup low-sodium vegetable broth (60ml)
- 1 tsp fresh basil, oregano, chopped (1g)
- Salt and pepper to taste

Instructions:

1. Preheat the oven to 375°F (190°C).
2. Roast bell peppers for 20–25 minutes, turning occasionally, until charred.Remove skins ,seeds.
3. Sauté onion in olive oil, then blend with roasted peppers, vegetable broth, and sautéed onion until smooth. Transfer sauce to a pan, add basil, oregano, salt, pepper, and simmer for 5 minutes.
4. Sauté spinach in olive oil until wilted.
5. In a baking dish, layer zucchini strips, ricotta, spinach, sauce, and mozzarella. Repeat layers, top with Parmesan, Italian seasoning, salt, and allspice. Bake for 30 minutes until golden and bubbly.

Nutritional Facts (Per Serving): Calories: 375 | Protein: 18g | Fat: 13g | Carbs: 15g | Fiber: 8g | Sodium: 450mg | Sugars: 7g

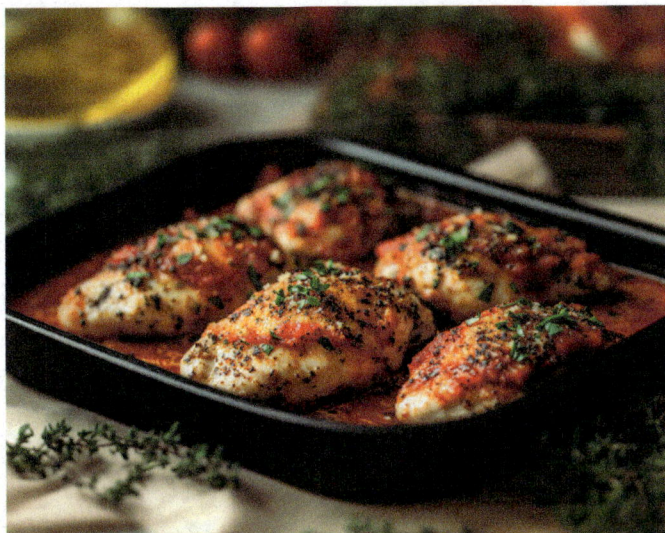

Baked chicken parmesan

Prep: 10 minutes | Cook: 25 minutes | Serves: 2

Ingredients:

- 4 boneless, skinless chicken thighs (300g)
- 1 tbsp olive oil (15ml)
- 1/2 cup low-fat cream (120ml)
- 1/4 cup low-sodium chicken broth (60ml)
- 1/4 cup grated Parmesan cheese (30g)
- 1/2 tsp dried thyme (1g)
- 1 tbsp olive oil (15ml)
- Salt and allspice to taste
- Fresh parsley, chopped (for garnish)

Instructions:

1. Preheat the oven to 375°F (190°C).
2. Dip chicken breasts in egg white, then coat with breadcrumbs seasoned with salt and allspice.
3. Heat olive oil in a pan over medium heat and sear the chicken until golden on both sides.
4. Place the chicken in a baking dish, top with marinara sauce, mozzarella, and Parmesan cheese.
5. Bake for 20-25 minutes, until cheese is melted and chicken is cooked through.

Nutritional Facts (Per Serving): Calories: 380 | Protein: 19g | Fat: 14g | Carbs: 18g | Fiber: 7g | Sodium: 450mg | Sugars: 7g

Meal Plans and Shopping Templates: Simplified for You

This cookbook includes a 30-day grocery shopping guide tailored for one person, designed to streamline your journey to an acid reflux-friendly diet. The guide focuses on fresh, high-quality ingredients, minimizing potential triggers and processed foods. Quantities are flexible, allowing you to adjust to your needs while enjoying balanced, soothing meals. Start eating comfortably and deliciously with ease!

Grocery Shopping List for 7-Day Meal Plan

Meat & Poultry:

- **Ground turkey** – 1 lb / 450 g (*Turkey Meatballs with Spaghetti Squash*)
- **Chicken breast (boneless, skinless)** – 2 lb / 900 g (*Egg Casserole with Chicken and Broccoli, Chicken and Spinach Zucchini Noodle Bake*)
- **Lamb (stew meat or chops)** – 1 lb / 450 g (*Braised Lamb with Rosemary and Vegetables*)

Fish & Seafood:

- **Salmon fillets** – 12 oz / 340 g (*Poached Salmon with Dill Sauce*)
- **Trout fillets** – 10 oz / 300 g (*Baked Trout with Almonds*)

Vegetables:

- **Spinach (fresh)** – 4 cups / 250 g (*Spinach and Ricotta Pancakes, Kiwi and Spinach Smoothie, Chicken and Spinach Zucchini Noodle Bake*)
- **Zucchini** – 3 large (*Vegetable Lasagna with Zucchini Noodles, Chicken and Spinach Zucchini Noodle Bake*)
- **Eggplant** – 2 medium (*Stuffed Eggplants Baked with Cheese Crust*)
- **Broccoli (florets)** – 2 cups / 150 g (*Egg Casserole with Chicken and Broccoli*)
- **Butternut squash (cubed)** – 1 cup / 150 g (*Pumpkin Sage Pasta*)
- **Cauliflower (florets)** – 1 head / 600 g (*Creamy Cauliflower Soup*)
- **Mushrooms (fresh)** – 2 cups / 150 g (*Vegetable Lasagna with Zucchini Noodles*)
- **Brussels sprouts** – 2 cups / 150 g (*Warm Brussels Sprouts and Bacon Salad*)
- **Carrots** – 2 medium (*Minestrone Soup*)
- **Celery** – 2 stalks (*Minestrone Soup*)
- **Onions (yellow)** – 3 medium (*Stuffed Eggplants Baked with Cheese Crust, Minestrone Soup*)
- **Garlic** – 1 bulb (*Various recipes*)
- **Fresh dill** – 1 bunch (*Poached Salmon with Dill Sauce*)

Fruits:

- **Bananas** – 2 large (*Pear Ginger Oatmeal*)
- **Blueberries** – 1 cup / 150 g (*Blueberry and Almond Energy Bites*)
- **Kiwi** – 3 large (*Kiwi and Spinach Smoothie, Kiwi and Chia Seed Parfait*)
- **Apples (sweet)** – 3 medium (*Apple and Cinnamon Yogurt Dip*)
- **Pears** – 2 medium (*Pear Ginger Oatmeal*)

Grains & Bread:

- **Quinoa** – 1 cup / 180 g (*Chickpea and Quinoa Pilaf, Quinoa and Vegetable Stew*)
- **Rolled oats** – 1 cup / 90 g (*Pear Ginger Oatmeal*)
- **Whole-grain pasta** – 2 cups / 200 g (*Pumpkin Sage Pasta, Herb Chicken Pasta Primavera*)
- **Whole-grain lasagna sheets** – 6 sheets (*Vegetable Lasagna with Zucchini Noodles*)

Dairy & Eggs:

- **Ricotta cheese** – 8 oz / 225 g (*Spinach and Ricotta Pancakes*)
- **Cottage cheese** – 8 oz / 225 g (*Pancakes with Cottage Cheese, Vanilla, and Raisins with Yogurt Sauce*)
- **Parmesan cheese** – 4 oz / 115 g (*Pumpkin Sage Pasta, Herb Chicken Pasta Primavera*)
- **Mozzarella cheese (fresh)** – 4 oz / 115 g (*Vegetable*

Lasagna with Zucchini Noodles)

- **Eggs (large)** – 18 (*Egg Casserole with Chicken and Broccoli, Ricotta and Herb-Stuffed Eggs, Pancakes with Cottage Cheese, Vanilla, and Raisins with Yogurt Sauce*)

Nuts, Seeds & Nut Butter:

- **Almonds (whole)** – ½ cup / 75 g (*Blueberry and Almond Energy Bites*)
- **Chia seeds** – ¼ cup / 40 g (*Kiwi and Chia Seed Parfait*)
- **Pumpkin seeds** – ¼ cup / 40 g (*Pumpkin and Sage Spread*)

Pantry Staples:

- **Olive oil (extra virgin)** – 1 bottle (*Various recipes*)
- **Honey** – 2 tbsp (*Oatmeal Honey Muffins*)
- **Pumpkin puree** – 1 small can (*Pumpkin Sage Pasta*)
- **Vegetable broth (low sodium)** – 2 cups / 500 ml (*Creamy Cauliflower Soup, Minestrone Soup*)
- **All-purpose flour** – 1 cup / 120 g (*Oatmeal Honey Muffins, Pancakes with Cottage Cheese, Vanilla, and Raisins with Yogurt Sauce*)

Meat & Poultry:

- **Ground turkey** – 1 lb / 450 g (*Mini Chicken Meatballs*)
- **Chicken breast (boneless, skinless)** – 1.5 lb / 675 g (*Spinach and Mushroom Stuffed Chicken Breast, Mediterranean Chicken Wrap*)
- **Turkey breast slices** – 8 oz / 225 g (*Turkey and Cranberry Pinwheels*)
- **Lamb chops** – 1 lb / 450 g (*Lamb Chops with Sweet Potato Mash*)
- **Pork tenderloin** – 1 lb / 450 g (*Stuffed Pork Tenderloin*)
- **Eggs** – 18 large (*Scrambled Eggs with Zucchini, Thin Egg Pancakes with Vegetable Filling, Eggs Baked in Small Buns with Bell Peppers*)

Fish & Seafood:

- **Haddock fillets** – 12 oz / 340 g (*Haddock Cutlets with Cabbage Salad and Cheese Sauce*)
- **Mackerel fillets** – 10 oz / 300 g (*Grilled Mackerel with Cucumber Salad*)

Vegetables:

- **Spinach (fresh)** – 4 cups / 250 g (*Spinach and Artichoke Dip, Spinach and Artichoke Risotto, Spinach and Mushroom Stuffed Chicken Breast*)
- **Zucchini** – 3 large (*Scrambled Eggs with Zucchini, Farro and Roasted Vegetable Bowl*)
- **Sweet potato** – 2 medium (*Lamb Chops with Sweet Potato Mash*)
- **Cabbage (shredded)** – 2 cups / 150 g (*Haddock Cutlets with Cabbage Salad and Cheese Sauce*)
- **Bell peppers (red or yellow)** – 3 medium (*Eggs Baked in Small Buns with Bell Peppers, Grilled Vegetable Fajitas with Cashew Cheese Sauce*)
- **Mushrooms (fresh)** – 2 cups / 150 g (*Mushroom Barley Stew, Spinach and Mushroom Stuffed Chicken Breast*)
- **Cauliflower (florets)** – 1 head / 600 g (*Cauliflower and Lentil Shepherd's Pie*)
- **Brussels sprouts** – 2 cups / 150 g (*Roasted Brussels Sprouts with Balsamic Glaze*)
- **Cucumber** – 1 large (*Grilled Mackerel with Cucumber Salad*)
- **Carrots** – 2 medium (*Green Pea and Basil Soup, Mushroom Barley Stew*)
- **Celery** – 2 stalks (*Turkey and Wild Rice Soup*)
- **Garlic** – 1 bulb (*Various recipes*)
- **Basil (fresh)** – 1 bunch (*Basil and Ricotta Spread, Green Pea and Basil Soup*)

Fruits:

- **Bananas** – 2 large (*Maple Pecan Quinoa Porridge*)
- **Berries (blueberries, strawberries)** – 1.5 cups / 225 g (*Cottage Cheese with Seasonal Berries and Sour Cream Sauce, Cakes with Whipped Cottage Cheese Mousse and Seasonal Berries*)
- **Pears** – 2 medium (*Vanilla Chia and Flax Porridge*)
- **Apples (sweet)** – 2 medium (*Turkey and Cranberry Pinwheels*)
- **Pumpkin puree** – 1 small can (*Pumpkin Spice Waffles*)

Grains & Bread:

- **Quinoa** – 1 cup / 180 g (*Maple Pecan Quinoa Porridge, Turkey and Wild Rice Soup*)
- **Farro** – 1 cup / 180 g (*Farro and Roasted Vegetable Bowl*)
- **Rice (wild)** – 1 cup / 180 g (*Turkey and Wild Rice Soup*)
- **Whole-grain wraps** – 2 medium (*Mediterranean Chicken Wrap*)

Dairy & Eggs:

- **Ricotta cheese** – 8 oz / 225 g (*Spinach and Artichoke Risotto, Basil and Ricotta Spread*)
- **Cottage cheese** – 8 oz / 225 g (*Cottage Cheese with Seasonal Berries and Sour Cream Sauce*)
- **Parmesan cheese** – 6 oz / 170 g (*Pea and Parmesan Risotto, Spinach and Artichoke Risotto*)
- **Cheddar cheese (shredded)** – 4 oz / 115 g (*Cauliflower and Lentil Shepherd's Pie*)

Nuts, Seeds & Nut Butter:

- **Pecans (chopped)** – ½ cup / 75 g (*Maple Pecan Quinoa Porridge*)
- **Chia seeds** – ¼ cup / 40 g (*Vanilla Chia and Flax Porridge*)

Pantry Staples:

- **Olive oil (extra virgin)** – 1 bottle (*Various recipes*)
- **Vegetable broth (low sodium)** – 2 cups / 500 ml (*Green Pea and Basil Soup, Mushroom Barley Stew*)
- **Cashew cheese** – 4 oz / 115 g (*Grilled Vegetable Fajitas with Cashew Cheese Sauce*)
- **Honey** – 2 tbsp (*Vanilla Chia and Flax Porridge*)

Grocery Shopping List for 15-21 Day Meal Plan

Meat & Poultry:

- **Ground turkey** – 1 lb / 450 g (*Amaranth Veggie Patties*)
- **Turkey sausage** – 8 oz / 225 g (*Turkey Sausage and Egg Muffins*)
- **Chicken breast (boneless, skinless)** – 1 lb / 450 g (*Honey Mustard Chicken with Roasted Brussels Sprouts, Herb Chicken Pasta Primavera*)
- **Cooked turkey slices** – 6 oz / 175 g (*Turkey and Cranberry Pinwheels*)
- **Eggs** – 18 large (*Egg White and Vegetable Wrap, Ricotta and Herb-Stuffed Eggs, Bruschetta with Boiled Eggs*)

Fish & Seafood:

- **Shrimp (peeled and deveined)** – 10 oz / 300 g (*Shrimp and Avocado Salad*)
- **Salmon fillets** – 10 oz / 300 g (*Poached Salmon with Dill Sauce*)

Vegetables:

- **Spinach (fresh)** – 4 cups / 250 g (*Spinach and Ricotta Pancakes, Spinach and Feta Stuffed Mushrooms, Zucchini Noodles with Pesto*)
- **Zucchini** – 3 large (*Zucchini Noodles with Pesto, Herb-Roasted Turkey with Vegetables*)
- **Brussels sprouts** – 2 cups / 150 g (*Honey Mustard Chicken with Roasted Brussels Sprouts*)
- **Cabbage (shredded)** – 1 cup / 150 g (*Fish Lettuce Wraps with Cabbage Slaw*)
- **Asparagus (fresh)** – 1 bunch / 300 g (*Bruschetta with Boiled Eggs, Soft Cheese, and Asparagus*)
- **Mushrooms (fresh)** – 2 cups / 150 g (*Spinach and Feta Stuffed Mushrooms, Mushroom and Asparagus Risotto*)
- **Carrots** – 2 medium (*Pumpkin and Sage Mashed Soup, Minestrone Soup*)
- **Celery** – 2 stalks (*Minestrone Soup*)
- **Apples (sweet)** – 2 medium (*Cucumber and Apple Smoothie*)
- **Garlic** – 1 bulb (*Various recipes*)
- **Fresh dill** – 1 bunch (*Poached Salmon with Dill Sauce*)

Fruits:

- **Kiwi** – 3 large (*Kiwi Poppy Seed Waffles*)
- **Blueberries (fresh or frozen)** – 1 cup / 150 g (*Blueberries Vanilla Millet Porridge*)
- **Bananas (ripe)** – 2 medium (*Low-Acid Banana Cake*)
- **Avocados** – 2 large (*Shrimp and Avocado Salad*)
- **Cucumber** – 1 large (*Cucumber and Apple Smoothie*)

Grains & Bread:

- **Quinoa** – 1 cup / 180 g (*Chickpea and Quinoa Pilaf*)
- **Millet (uncooked)** – 1 cup / 180 g (*Blueberries Vanilla Millet Porridge*)
- **Pasta (whole-grain)** – 1 cup / 180 g (*Herb Chicken Pasta Primavera*)
- **Whole-grain wraps** – 2 medium (*Fish Lettuce Wraps with Cabbage Slaw*)

Dairy & Eggs:

- **Ricotta cheese** – 8 oz / 225 g (*Spinach and Ricotta Pancakes, Ricotta and Herb-Stuffed Eggs*)
- **Feta cheese** – 6 oz / 170 g (*Spinach and Feta Stuffed Mushrooms*)
- **Cream cheese (low-fat)** – 4 oz / 115 g (*Herb Cream Cheese*)

- **Parmesan cheese** – 4 oz / 115 g (*Mushroom and Asparagus Risotto*)
- **Soft cheese (e.g., Brie or Camembert)** – 4 oz / 115 g (*Bruschetta with Boiled Eggs, Soft Cheese, and Asparagus*)

Nuts, Seeds & Nut Butter:

- **Poppy seeds** – 2 tbsp / 30 g (*Kiwi Poppy Seed Waffles*)

Pantry Staples:

- **Olive oil (extra virgin)** – 1 bottle (*Various recipes*)
- **Vegetable broth (low sodium)** – 3 cups / 750 ml (*Minestrone Soup, Pumpkin and Sage Mashed Soup*)
- **Pumpkin puree** – 1 small can (*Pumpkin and Sage Mashed Soup, Pumpkin and Coconut Pudding*)
- **Coconut milk (canned)** – 1 cup / 250 ml (*Pumpkin and Coconut Pudding*)
- **Honey** – 2 tbsp (*Cucumber and Apple Smoothie, Kiwi Poppy Seed Waffles*)
- **Pesto sauce** – 4 oz / 115 g (*Zucchini Noodles with Pesto*)

Meat & Poultry:

- **Ground beef** – 1 lb / 450 g (*Lean Beef and Lamb Meatloaf with Herbs and Vegetables*)
- **Ground lamb** – 1 lb / 450 g (*Lean Beef and Lamb Meatloaf with Herbs and Vegetables*)
- **Chicken breast (boneless, skinless)** – 2 lb / 900 g (*Egg Casserole with Chicken and Broccoli, Chicken and Mushroom Casserole*)
- **Chicken thighs** – 1 lb / 450 g (*Turkey and Spinach Mini Rolls*)
- **Ground turkey** – 1 lb / 450 g (*Mini Chicken Meatballs*)
- **Turkey slices** – 8 oz / 225 g (*Turkey and Spinach Mini Rolls*)

Fish & Seafood:

- **Calamari (cleaned, whole)** – 12 oz / 340 g (*Stuffed Calamari with Spinach-Lemon Dressing*)

Vegetables:

- **Spinach (fresh)** – 5 cups / 300 g (*Vanilla Chia and Flax Porridge, Stuffed Calamari with Spinach-Lemon Dressing, Grilled Vegetable Fajitas with Cashew Cheese Sauce, Chicken and Mushroom Casserole*)
- **Zucchini** – 3 large (*Farro and Roasted Vegetable Bowl, Grilled Vegetable Fajitas with Cashew Cheese Sauce*)
- **Eggplant** – 2 medium (*Stuffed Eggplants Baked with Cheese Crust*)
- **Brussels sprouts** – 2 cups / 150 g (*Warm Brussels Sprouts and Bacon Salad*)
- **Cauliflower (florets)** – 1 head / 600 g (*Cauliflower Rice Bake*)
- **Mushrooms (fresh)** – 2 cups / 150 g (*Baked Mushroom Fritters with Sour Cream Sauce, Chicken and Mushroom Casserole*)
- **Broccoli (florets)** – 2 cups / 150 g (*Asian-Style Boiled Lenten Beef and Broccoli with Wild Rice*)

- **Peas (fresh or frozen)** – 1 cup / 150 g (*Green Pea and Basil Soup*)
- **Carrots** – 3 medium (*Quinoa and Vegetable Stew, Green Pea and Basil Soup*)
- **Celery** – 2 stalks (*Quinoa and Vegetable Stew*)
- **Bell peppers (red or yellow)** – 2 medium (*Egg White and Vegetable Wrap, Grilled Vegetable Fajitas with Cashew Cheese Sauce*)
- **Garlic** – 1 bulb (*Various recipes*)
- **Basil (fresh)** – 1 bunch (*Green Pea and Basil Soup*)

Fruits:

- **Bananas (ripe)** – 3 medium (*Banana Almond Buckwheat Porridge*)
- **Blueberries (fresh or frozen)** – 1 cup / 150 g (*Cakes with Whipped Cottage Cheese Mousse and Seasonal Berries*)
- **Kiwi** – 3 large (*Kiwi and Spinach Smoothie, Kiwi and Chia Seed Parfait*)
- **Apples (sweet)** – 2 medium (*Apple and Cinnamon Yogurt Dip*)

Grains & Bread:

- **Buckwheat groats** – 1 cup / 180 g (*Banana Almond Buckwheat Porridge*)
- **Quinoa** – 1 cup / 180 g (*Quinoa and Vegetable Stew*)
- **Farro** – 1 cup / 180 g (*Farro and Roasted Vegetable Bowl*)
- **Wild rice** – 1 cup / 180 g (*Asian-Style Boiled Lenten Beef and Broccoli with Wild Rice*)

Dairy & Eggs:

- **Cottage cheese** – 8 oz / 225 g (*Cakes with Whipped Cottage Cheese Mousse and*

Seasonal Berries)

- **Feta cheese** – 4 oz / 115 g (*Stuffed Eggplants Baked with Cheese Crust*)
- **Parmesan cheese** – 4 oz / 115 g (*Herb Chicken Pasta Primavera*)
- **Cheddar cheese (shredded)** – 4 oz / 115 g (*Cauliflower Rice Bake*)
- **Greek yogurt (plain)** – 8 oz / 225 g (*Apple and Cinnamon Yogurt Dip*)
- **Eggs** – 18 large (*Egg Casserole with Chicken*

and Broccoli, Egg White and Vegetable Wrap, Mini Chicken Meatballs)

Nuts, Seeds & Nut Butter:

- **Chia seeds** – ¼ cup / 40 g (*Vanilla Chia and Flax Porridge, Kiwi and Chia Seed Parfait*)

Pantry Staples:

- **Olive oil (extra virgin)** – 1 bottle (*Various recipes*)
- **Vegetable broth (low**

sodium) – 2 cups / 500 ml (*Quinoa and Vegetable Stew, Green Pea and Basil Soup*)

- **Honey** – 2 tbsp (*Kiwi and Spinach Smoothie, Banana Almond Buckwheat Porridge*)
- **Cashew cheese** – 4 oz / 115 g (*Grilled Vegetable Fajitas with Cashew Cheese Sauce*)
- **Pumpkin puree** – 1 small can (*Pumpkin Spice Waffles*)

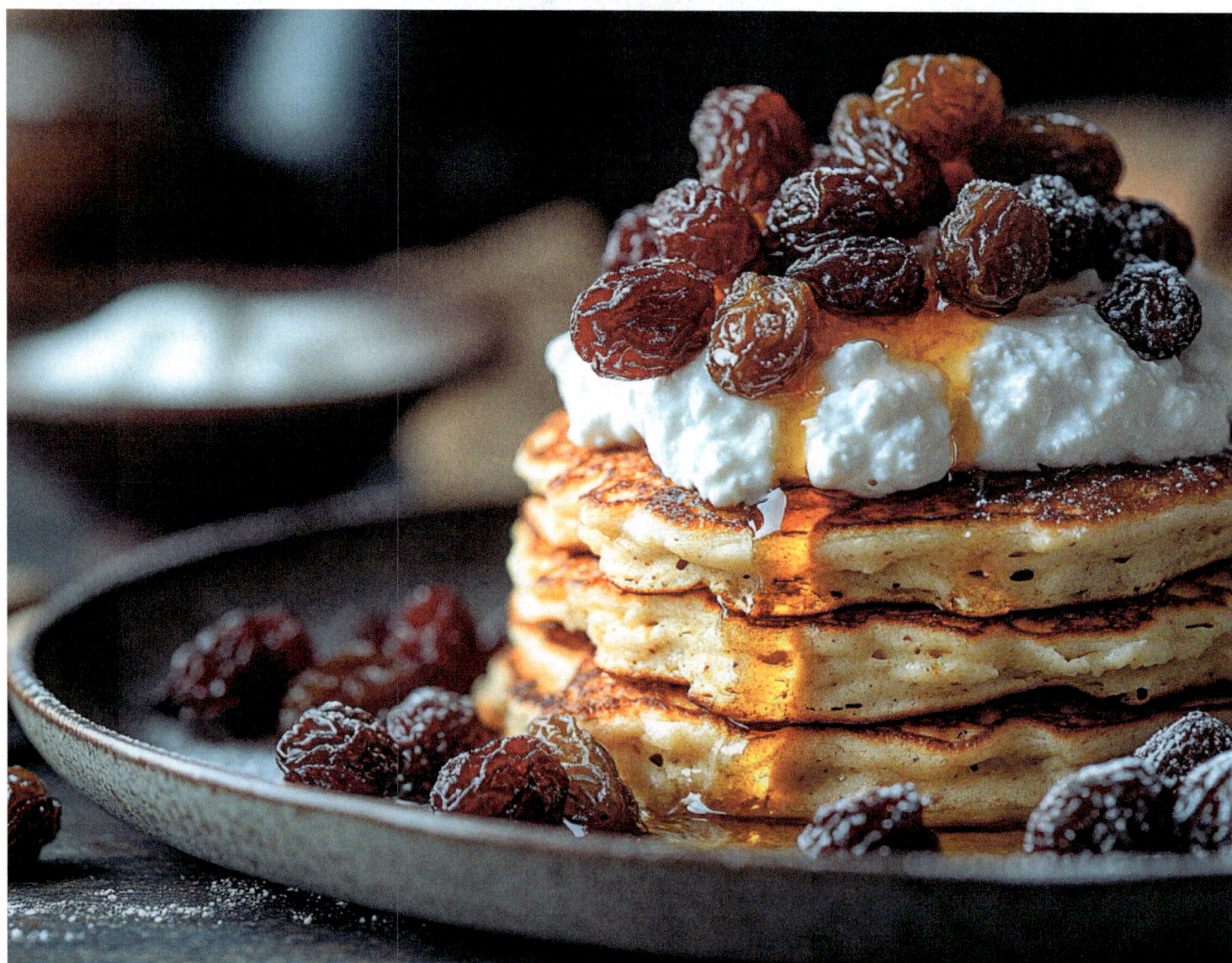

APPENDIX MEASUREMENT CONVERSION CHART

VOLUME EQUIVALENTS (DRY)

US STANDARD	METRIC (APPROXIMATE)
1/8 teaspoon	0.5 mL
1/4 teaspoon	1 mL
1/2 teaspoon	2 mL
3/4 teaspoon	4 mL
1 teaspoon	5 mL
1 tablespoon	15 mL
1/4 cup	59 mL
1/2 cup	118 mL
3/4 cup	177 mL
1 cup	235 mL
2 cups	475 mL
3 cups	700 mL
4 cups	1 L

WEIGHT EQUIVALENTS

US STANDARD	METRIC (APPROXIMATE)
1 ounce	28 g
2 ounces	57 g
5 ounces	142 g
10 ounces	284 g
15 ounces	425 g
16 ounces	455 g
(1 pound)	680 g
1.5 pounds	907 g

VOLUME EQUIVALENTS (LIQUID)

US STANDARD	US STANDARD (OUNCES)	METRIC (APPROXIMATE)
2 tablespoons	1 fl.oz.	30 mL
1/4 cup	2 fl.oz.	60 mL
1/2 cup	4 fl.oz.	120 mL
1 cup	8 fl.oz.	240 mL
11/2 cup	12 fl.oz.	355 mL
2 cups or 1 pint	16 fl.oz.	475 mL
4 cups or 1 quart	32 fl.oz.	1 L
1 gallon	128 fl.oz.	4 L

TEMPERATURES EQUIVALENTS

FAHRENHEIT(F)	CELSIUS(C) (APPROXIMATE)
225 °F	107 °C
250 °F	120 °C
275 °F	135 °C
300 °F	150 °C
325 °F	160 °C
350 °F	180 °C
375 °F	190 °C
400 °F	205 °C
425 °F	220 °C
450 °F	235 °C
475 °F	245 °C
500 °F	260 °C

Printed in Dunstable, United Kingdom